PRACTICAL TIPS ON HOW TO LOSE WEIGHT IN 30 DAYS

DISCOVER YOUR POTENTIAL, LOSE WEIGHT, AND ADOPT A HEALTHIER LIFESTYLE WITH TRIED-AND-TRUE METHODS.

BONUS: RECIPES AND MEAL IDEAS TO KEEP YOU INSPIRED IN THE KITCHEN

BY ROSANNA B. HARRY

Copyright © 2024 Written by Rosanna B. Harry

Disclaimer Notice

This book's content is meant solely for informational and educational purposes. It is not meant to be a replacement for expert counsel or medical care. Any repercussions arising from the usage of the material included herein are not the responsibility of the author or publisher. Readers seeking assistance tailored to their situation should speak with a certified practitioner

ABOUT THE BOOK

Are you prepared to start losing weight and reach your health objectives in just thirty days? Your go-to resource for dropping extra weight and starting a healthy lifestyle is "Practical Tips on How to Lose Weight in 30 Days". This book will provide you with the tools to make long-lasting changes and accomplish your weight loss objectives in just one month. It is jam-packed with practical guidance, doable tactics, and professional insights.

Important Subjects Addressed:

Creating Realistic and Achievable Objectives: Discover how to create attainable objectives for your weight reduction that will keep you inspired and on track.

Knowing Your Body: Adjust your weight reduction strategy based on your understanding of the special requirements and metabolism of your body.

Learn about mindful eating practices, portion control, and meal planning as well as other useful advice for choosing healthier foods.

Including Physical Activity: Learn about efficient workout plans and methods for maintaining an active lifestyle all day long, even with a hectic schedule.

Lifestyle Adjustments: Make Lifestyle choices that will help you lose weight, such as controlling your stress levels, getting better sleep, and drinking plenty of water.

Tracking Progress: To ensure success, learn how to keep an eye on your progress and modify your weight-reduction plan as necessary**Overcoming Obstacles:** Recognize typical roadblocks and discover strategies to get past them, from managing cravings to maintaining motivation while hitting a slump.

Reiterating positive habits and behaviors for sustained success, celebrate your accomplishments and significant life events.

Who Can Benefit: "Practical Tips on How to Lose Weight in 30 Days" is your go-to resource for attaining significant results in a short period, whether you're trying to kickstart your weight loss journey, overcome a plateau, or simply adopt healthier habits. This book gives you the tools you need to take charge of your health and change your life in just 30 days, along with useful advice and doable tactics.

In conclusion, are you prepared to start the journey to a happier, healthier version of yourself? Explore "Practical Tips on How to Lose Weight in 30 Days" to start your journey toward improved health and well-being. If you have the correct tools, commitment, and determination, you may make long-lasting changes that go well beyond the next 30 days and reach your weight loss objectives.

ABOUT THE AUTHOR

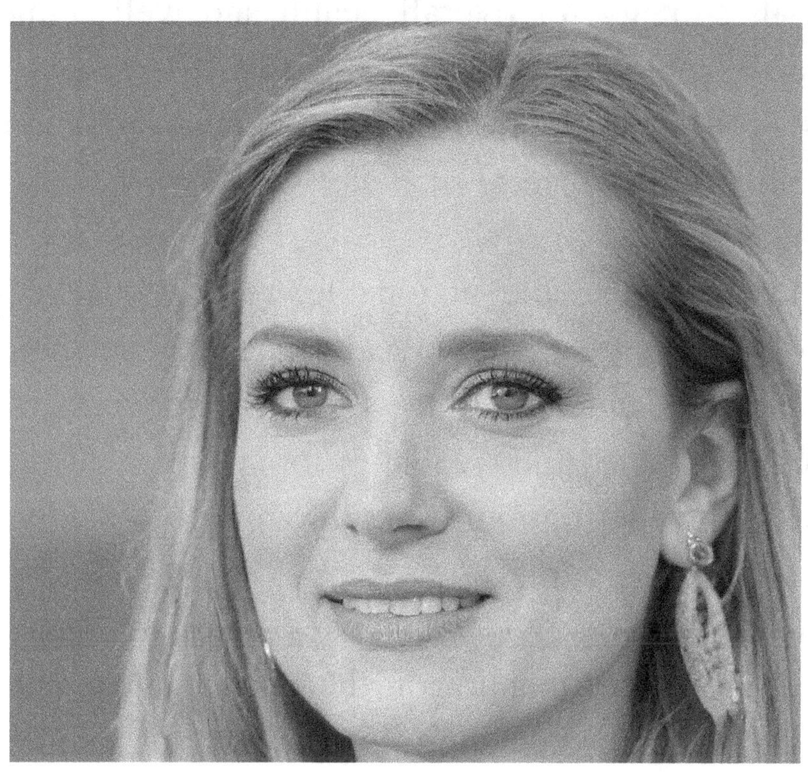

To uplift and enable others to live their best lives, Rosanna B. Harry is an ardent supporter of health and wellbeing. Rosanna has devoted her professional life to assisting individuals in reaching their health objectives by using doable, long-term solutions. She has a background in both fitness and nutrition.

Motivated by her own experience overcoming health obstacles and reaching her goal weight, Rosanna has gained a profound comprehension of the intricacies involved in weight reduction and the significance of adopting a comprehensive approach to well-being. She has developed her knowledge in areas including stress management, exercise, healthy eating, and behavior modification from her personal experiences and in-depth research.

Rosanna's weight loss strategy is based on empathy, comprehension, and a dedication to accepting individuals for who they are. She thinks that there is no one-size-fits-all strategy for overall health and well-being because each person is different. Rather, Rosanna stresses the need to figure out what suits you and implement sustainable lifestyle adjustments that promote long-term success.

Rosanna is committed to giving people actionable, research-backed information so they can take charge of their health and change their lives. She is a certified nutrition coach and fitness fanatic. She works to make healthy living approachable and realistic for people of all backgrounds and fitness levels through her writing, speaking engagements, and online coaching programs.

Rosanna enjoys being outside, experimenting in the kitchen with new dishes, and working out at the gym when she's not encouraging people to lead healthier lives. She is a respected source of inspiration and advice in the health and wellness world because of her infectious enthusiasm for life and sincere desire to help others.

TABLE OF CONTENTS

CHAPTER 6: KNOWLEDGE OF CALORIES: HOW MUCH IS SUFFICIENT?

- Determining The Optimal Balance Between Calories Burned And Consumed.
- Avoid Common Mistakes That Could Make Your Weight Loss Efforts More Difficult.

CHAPTER 7: MOVING YOUR BODY: SELECTING ENJOYABLE EXERCISE

- Trying Out Different Types Of Exercise To Determine What Works For You.

CHAPTER 8: MANAGING STRESS AND EMOTIONAL CONSUMPTION

- Determining The Reasons Behind Emotional Eating
- Using Techniques For Relaxation To Reduce Stress
- Developing Healthy Coping Mechanisms Without Food

CHAPTER 9: PRIORITIZING SLEEP FOR EFFECTIVE WEIGHT LOSS

- Understanding The Connection Between Sleep And Losing Weight.
- Making A Nighttime Routine To Improve The Quality Of Your Sleep
- Changing Your Sleeping Surroundings To Improve Your Quality Of Sleep

CHAPTER 10: GETTING PAST CHALLENGES

- Handling The Irksome Periods When Your Weight Loss Stops
- Trying New Strategies To Quicken Your Progress
- Keeping Motivation And Optimism In The Face Of Difficulty

CHAPTER 11: GETTING HELP WHEN REQUIRED

- Mentioning Support From Friends And Family, Companions, Or Web Gatherings.
- Finding a Responsibility Accomplice
- What Kinds of Treatment Are Ideal?

CHAPTER 12: OVERSEEING HESITANCE AND DISAPPOINTMENTS

- Making Plans For Defeating Enticements And Wants
- Recognizing Blunders And Using Them As Opportunities For Development.

CHAPTER 13: RESPECTING YOUR PROSPERITY
- Sorting Out Some Way To Treat Yourself When You Achieve Objectives.
- Committing To A Happier, Healthier Lifestyle Long-term
- Making The Shift From Weight Reduction To Maintenance
- Techniques For Avoiding Relapse And Maintaining Focus

CONCLUSION: YOUR PATH TO A HEALTHIER LIFESTYLE
- Resolving To Pursue Ongoing Development And Personal Advancement
- Considering The Lessons You've Learned And The Adjustments You've Made.
- Motivating People To Set Out On Their Path To Improved Health
- Tools For Monitoring Your Development And Creating New Objectives.

RECIPES AND MEAL IDEAS TO KEEP YOU INSPIRED IN THE KITCHEN
- Breakfast Treats:
- Lunch Ideas:
- Ideas for Dinner:
- Filling Snacks:
- Nutritious Dessert Treats:
- Winners of Meal Prep:

GLOSSARY PAGE

CHAPTER 1: OVERVIEW AND OBJECTIVE ESTABLISHMENT

Introduction

This is "Practical Tips on How to Lose Weight in 30 Days." You're going to start a journey to a better, healthier version of yourself over the next thirty days. The purpose of this book is to give you useful guidance, doable suggestions, and tried-and-true methods to assist you successfully and long-term lose weight.

In the fast-paced world of today, it's simple to put convenience over health. But you can establish lifelong beneficial habits by setting out just thirty days to concentrate on your well-being. This book will help you at every stage, whether your goal is to lose weight, increase your energy, or just enhance your general health.

You will not only shed pounds but also regain your energy, vitality, and sense of well-being by adopting new lifestyle practices, consistent exercise, and a balanced diet. Now let's get started on your road of change to become a happier, healthier version of yourself!

Before starting your 30-day weight loss journey, you must set attainable and well-defined goals. Setting goals gives you a path to achievement and keeps you motivated and focused along the way. Here are some pointers on making truly impactful goals:

Be Specific: Rather than establishing nebulous objectives such as "lose weight," specify exactly what you hope to accomplish. For instance, set a goal to drop a specific amount of weight or inches, or resolve to wear a particular size of clothes.

Make Them Measurable: To monitor your success, your goals must be quantifiable. Divide your overarching objective into more manageable checkpoints that you can commemorate along the route.

Establish Reasonable Expectations: It's important to push yourself, but it's equally important to establish achievable objectives. Being honest with yourself about your existing lifestyle, commitments, and health state will help you determine what you can do in thirty days.

Establish a Deadline: Give yourself a deadline to meet your objectives. A decent beginning point for your weight loss journey is thirty days, although you are welcome to modify this to suit your goals and tastes.

Put Your Goals in Writing: Writing down your objectives will help you feel more committed to reaching them and will give them a more tangible sense. To keep them visible and in the forefront of your mind, think about writing them down in a notebook or making a vision board.

Maintain Flexibility: Setting objectives is important, but you also need to be adaptive and flexible. Unexpected obstacles are a common part of life, so be ready to modify your plans as necessary and practice self-compassion as you go.

You'll position yourself for success and create the groundwork for a fruitful 30-day weight loss journey by establishing specific, attainable goals. Thus, give it some thought and make a commitment to achieving your goals for the next thirty days. This is something you can handle!

Defining Your Weight Loss Objectives

When attempting to reduce weight, setting objectives aids in controlling expectations, tracking advancement, and maintaining focus. However, choosing the appropriate goals can be challenging given the wealth of information available online. We've put together some goal-setting advice and provided links to tools to support you in reaching your objectives in order to assist you on your weight reduction journey.

How to make reasonable objectives for weight reduction
It is crucial to determine whether you are now a healthy weight before setting any weight loss goals. You may accomplish this by using a BMI calculator. It will calculate a score that falls into different categories based on your height and weight. Instead of focusing on weight loss, if you fall into the healthy weight range and are neither overweight nor obese, consider keeping your current weight. One of the best things you can do for your health is to maintain a healthy weight, which lowers your chance of developing a number of diseases, including diabetes, heart disease, and some types of cancer.

Please be aware that there are some limitations to BMI, and it's critical to be aware of these before beginning a weight loss program.

The BMI divisions:
A healthy weight ranges from 18.5 to 24.9.
25 to 29.9 is considered overweight.
Obese: between 30 and 39.9.
A BMI of 40 or higher indicates extreme obesity.

If you are obese or overweight, your first goal should be to reduce a modest amount of weight (five percent is a reasonable figure to strive for). For instance, if you weigh 15 stone, this appears to be 10.5 pounds.
Reducing five percent of your body weight can have positive effects on your health, including lowering blood pressure and the risk of diabetes. Consider aiming for 10% if you need to lose a lot of weight, but don't forget to celebrate your accomplishment and keep yourself motivated when you reach the 5% level!

Lose one to two pounds every week.
Most doctors agree that it's safe to aim for weekly weight loss of one to two pounds. This equates to 500–1,000 less calories per day on average than what you need to consume to stay at your present weight. If you need assistance calculating a calorie deficit, speak with your physician or a dietician.

Depending on exercise levels, the recommended daily calorie intake for males and women is 2,500 and 2,000, respectively. In addition to offering examples of balanced meals, our healthy eating guide is a helpful resource for learning about appropriate portion proportions.

Think about the immediate

Small goals helped dieters accomplish long-term objectives, according to a research. The overall number of pounds you wish to drop when beginning a weight loss program may seem overwhelming. If you set tiny objectives, such as tracking your daily intake and figuring out how much weight you need to lose each week, you're more likely to "meet subsequent goals, week to week and month to month."

Make SMART objectives for weight loss.

SMART goals make it easier for certain people to create and accomplish their objectives. SMART objectives are:

Particular: What precisely are you hoping to achieve?
Measurable: How will you determine when it has been completed?
Achievable: how will you get there and is it feasible given other circumstances?
Relevant: Is it important to you? Does it seem like the appropriate moment?
Time-bound: what is the start date and end date?
A SMART weight loss goal would look something like this: "Join a local exercise class and cut back on calories to lose one stone of weight in 12 months." My need to reduce my blood pressure and my want to engage in more activities with my grandchildren serve as my motivation.

Monitor your progress with weight loss.

To stay motivated, it's critical to monitor weight loss. You can use an outdated chart on paper or one of the many free weight tracking applications available! There are several methods for determining weight reduction besides just keeping track of weight. For instance, your sense of wellness may have increased, your clothes may fit better, or you may notice changes in certain body measurements, such as those of your waist, hips, and thighs.

Establish activity objectives.

Setting objectives for your activities can also help you stay motivated and reap some of the benefits of reducing weight. They can assist you in achieving your objectives more quickly. Possible objectives for an activity could be:

Performing 30 minutes of physical activity, such as walking or swimming, five days a week

Completing your neighborhood 5k Parkrun

enrolling in a neighborhood fitness program

In app challenges, like walking or running 100 kilometers every month

Understanding The Factors That Influence Loss of Weight

Have you always thought that losing weight is simple and only requires cutting less on food and increasing exercise to burn off more calories than you take in? This is undoubtedly what many nutritionists and fitness gurus advise us to do.

The variables influencing weight loss are more intricate, though.

If you're following a diet and exercise routine but finding it difficult to drop the weight or maintain the weight you do lose, there may be additional factors at play.

Let's take a closer look at them.

1. GENES

Why is it that some people are destined to suffer with weight gain and, consequently, attempt to reduce weight throughout their lives, while others may eat anything they want without gaining weight?

Our weight is essentially governed by three factors: the number of calories we burn, store, and consume. This is explained in the article. However, from the time of conception onward, a combination of our genes and environment have a significant impact on these factors.

More than 400 genes have been found by scientists to have some bearing on body weight to yet. Our appetite, satiety (the duration for which we feel full), metabolism, food cravings, body-fat distribution, and even our emotional connection to food—such as eating during stressful situations or having a tendency to develop eating disorders—are all influenced by these genes.

According to recent studies, there is a wide range in the degree to which our genes influence weight gain or reduction. Genetic influence on the propensity to be overweight or obese is thought to be as low as 25% in some individuals and as high as 70–80% in others.

HOW CAN YOU DISCOVER IF THERE IS A POSSIBLE GROUND FOR YOUR WEIGHT LOSS?
Speak with a physician who can examine your unique situation in order to ascertain whether your genes are impacting your weight reduction.

However, generally speaking, if you fit into any of the following criteria, you may be genetically predisposed to obesity:

You've spent the most of your life being overweight.

If one or both of your parents or other near blood relatives are severely overweight, there is an 80% hereditary probability that the child will also be obese if both parents are obese, according to a Harvard article.

You follow a rigorous low-calorie diet for several months and exercise frequently, yet you still find it difficult to lose weight.

Your genes might only have a modest impact on your ability to lose weight if you belong to any of the following groups:

Food availability directly affects and is correlated with your weight.

When you maintain a modest diet and exercise routine, you can lose weight.

You can lose weight again by changing your diet and activity level after gaining it during the holidays or during stressful times.

If you don't move much and you can consume foods high in calories without gaining weight, it's likely that you have a low genetic propensity for obesity.

2. ETHNICITY OR RACE

An increasing amount of research suggests that your ethnicity may have an impact on your weight, influencing both how quickly you gain weight and how simple it is to lose it.

Studies show that body fat tends to build closer to the center of our bodies around the age of thirty, and it also continues to climb steadily after that.
Data from the US Centers for Disease Control and Prevention (CDC) support this, but they also show how socioeconomic and ethnic factors—such as income levels, upbringing, access to healthcare, and place of residence—interplay in a complex way to influence obesity.

A growing number of medical professionals are interested in learning more about how race or ethnicity influences weight and how that will affect access to appropriate weight reduction support.

3. AGE

According to research, after the age of thirty, not only does body fat continue to rise consistently, but it also tends to accumulate closer to the center of our bodies and our internal organs. Up until the age of 65, women tend to gain weight more than males. After that, many of us lose some weight, usually as a result of a decline in muscle mass.

As we've seen above, obese children may struggle with their weight well into adulthood; this could be due in part to a strong genetic component.

4. GENDER/SEX

In the UK as a whole, 67% of men and 62% of women are classified as overweight or obese, according to NHS data. Men are more likely than women to be overweight (but not obese), whereas women are more likely than men to be obese (including morbidly obese).

In America, there is also a stated tendency toward increased rates of obesity in women; this trend is considerably more pronounced among African American and Hispanic women. It's crucial to acknowledge, though, that women in these groups frequently experience socioeconomic disparities, which may have an effect on their weight.

5. FOOD :

There's no denying that our ability to lose weight is influenced by the caliber and amount of our food. You may gain weight if you consume meals and drinks that are high in fat, sugar, and calories.

But this is where things might become complicated.

According to some experts, losing weight can be achieved by following the simple equation of burning more calories through activity than calories intake. So does this imply that you could lose weight even if you had 1,000 calories of cake rather than 1,000 calories of vegetables?

Though the human body is not so simple, they do!

Numerous meals and macronutrients have a wide range of effects on our hormones, appetite, cognitive function, and much more. For example, the numerous metabolic pathways they pass through influence how much of the energy in the food is consumed and how much is released as heat.

This is the reason it's critical to ensure that your diet is providing the maximum amount of nutrients, even if you're on a calorie-restricted one. Making sure you're eating the correct meals to assist your weight reduction is just one of the numerous benefits of adhering to a medically supervised weight loss program.

6. ACTIVITIES/EXERCISES IN PHYSIO

People who wish to lose weight frequently discuss nutrition and physical activity together. Our bodies burn a direct proportion of the calories we consume throughout the day based on the kinds of activities we engage in and how active we are.

Increasing your physical activity level is crucial for effective weight loss. When you do, though, it can be even more crucial for keeping your weight at a healthy level.

But maintaining an active lifestyle goes beyond controlling weight. It has been demonstrated that just 150 minutes a week of moderate-intensity aerobic activity—such as going for a brisk walk, riding in a casual setting, or playing with your kids in the park—can:

Lower elevated blood pressure

Lower your risk of heart attacks, strokes, type 2 diabetes, and a number of cancer types.

lessen the discomfort and handicap brought on by arthritis

Lower the risk of falls and osteoporosis

lessen the signs of worry and sadness

Once more, exercise in a medically supervised weight loss program is usually tailored to your objectives, level of fitness, and medical background.

7. YOUR HOME AND PLACE OF WORK

Socioeconomic factors may have an impact on your weight loss, as we have mentioned in a couple of the previous sections.

For instance, are there nice fresh fruit outlets and supermarket stores close to your home? Do you have easy access to any nearby parks or sports facilities by foot? Do you have extra money that you could spend on things like gym memberships or exercise classes?

What kind of catering services does your place of employment offer? Is it necessary to purchase fast food from a vending machine or is there a cafeteria that serves wholesome meals? Can you bring food from home into the office? Do you and your clients often go out to eat?

What sort of hours are you employed? Do you have a scheduled lunch break? Maybe you work shifts, so occasionally you eat at night and sleep during the day?

Your general health and well-being, as well as your weight, will be impacted by these and a plethora of other factors.

8. FAMILY CULTURE AND HABITS

Families, friendship groups, and broader society's attitudes toward body shape all have an inevitable impact on our commitment to weight loss, as well as how we view and react to weight gain.

You may develop similar behaviors later in life if your family members consume a lot of high-sugar meals or favor sedentary hobbies like playing computer games or watching TV.

In a similar vein, your experiences may differ if you come from a culture or religion that places a strong premium on particular food kinds or big family feasts. Additionally, opinions of body size and body image are influenced by culture from a young age. For instance, although some cultures value a smaller frame, others view being overweight as a sign of fertility, prosperity, health, and power.

A Psychology Today article outlined the relationship between income exercise and eating habits. Women in higher income brackets tend to be thinner than women in lower income brackets in the US and Europe, where thinness is still viewed as the "ideal" of beauty. This is because women in higher income brackets can afford services like personal training, gym memberships, spa treatments, nutritional support, and even food that is prepared and delivered by a strict diet. Additionally, they may have relatives and acquaintances that lead like lifestyles.

It's important to note that research in the American Journal of Public Health revealed that food portion sizes in America have increased significantly since the 1970s and currently surpass federal guidelines, which has a direct impact on the nation's rising obesity epidemic. Numerous other countries around the world, including the UK, have also noticed the same trends.

9. SLEEP

Getting enough sleep could be a key component of a successful weight loss plan.

Numerous studies have shown that individuals with four hours or less of sleep each night have altered metabolisms and increased appetites, especially for high-carbohydrate, calorie-dense foods.

One reason could be that the amount of sleep one gets influences the hormones ghrelin and leptin, which control appetite. The fact that exhaustion from sleep deprivation makes you feel less motivated to be active may also be a contributing factor.

Any action you can do to get a better night's sleep will probably help you reach your weight loss objectives and feel better overall.

10. MEDICATION AND MEDICAL CONDITIONS

Numerous medical diseases have the potential to either inhibit weight loss or induce weight gain. These include depression, menopause and other hormonal changes, Cushing's disease, metabolic syndrome, underactive thyroid, polycystic ovarian syndrome (PCOS), and others.

Furthermore, taking medicine for a variety of illnesses may make it more difficult to reduce weight. Medication for blood pressure reduction, diabetes, depression, epilepsy, and birth control are a few examples.

This is yet another reason that, at Medikaur, we support medically-led weight loss: if you are taking medication that is influencing your weight, you will have a medical expert by your side to support you.

When combined with a nutritious diet and way of life, certain drugs have also been demonstrated to help with weight loss. Again, if such medication is approved for this kind of use, it may be included in a medically supervised weight loss program.

11. ANXIETY

Finally, it's important to consider the possibility that stress is affecting your weight.

Research indicates that experiencing continuous stress in your life may lead to an increase in the stress hormone cortisol production in your body.

The hormone that alerts your body to the need to "fight or flight" is called cortisol. It also increases your hunger to ensure that you obtain the extra energy you need because it tricks your brain into thinking that it will be necessary for your survival.

You shouldn't have any serious negative effects if your cortisol levels rise momentarily, but persistent stress will keep your cortisol levels high and lead to the issues mentioned above.

According to other research, while you're under stress, your metabolism slows down (perhaps to save calories in case you have to sprint for it!). and you gain weight around your middle as a result of elevated cortisol levels.

You can lose weight more effectively by taking action to lower your stress levels.

CHAPTER 2: ASSESSING YOUR DAILY PRACTICES

The secret to a healthy lifestyle and improved weight control is nutritious food and a balanced way of living. Keeping a diet and weight journal, getting social support, and exercising frequently are some weight loss strategies.

The Centers for Disease Control and Prevention estimate that 93.3 million adult Americans (Trusted Source) were obese in 2015–2016. This figure represents 39.8% of the total population.

Being overweight raises the risk of heart disease, hypertension, and type 2 diabetes, among other major health issues.

Despite any benefits that its supporters may claim, crash diets are not a long-term answer. Making small, long-lasting, and advantageous lifestyle adjustments is crucial for safe and long-term weight loss.

Ten Suggestions For Effective Weight Loss

People who follow a few realistic steps can lose weight and keep it off. Among them are the following:

1. **Consume a wide variety of vibrant, nutrient-dense meals.**
Consume a healthy, diversified diet.
The basis of a person's diet should consist of nutritious meals and snacks. Making sure that each meal has 50% fruit and vegetables, 25% whole grains, and 25% protein is an easy method to build a meal plan. 25–30 grams of fiber should be consumed overall. Every day, Trusted Source (g).

Reduce your consumption of saturated fats, which are strongly associated with the risk of coronary heart disease, and get rid of trans fats from your diet.

As an alternative, people might eat unsaturated fats like polyunsaturated fatty acids (PUFA) and monounsaturated fatty acids (MUFA).

The foods listed below are nutritious and frequently high in nutrients:
Wholesome produce and fruits
Fish, lentils, seeds, and nuts
Whole grains, such as oats and brown rice

Items you should not consume include:
Eating rich red meats or processed meats that have added sugar, butter, or oils
baked products.
Bagels
White bread
Prepared meals

Sometimes cutting out particular items from the diet can result in a person lacking in important vitamins and minerals. A person pursuing a weight loss program can receive advice from a nutritionist, dietitian, or other healthcare professional on how to ensure they are getting adequate nutrients.

2. Maintain a food and weight log.

A key component of weight loss success is self-monitoring. To track every food item they eat each day, people can use a specialized website, mobile app, or paper journal. Another way they might track their development is by keeping a weekly weight log.

A person is far more likely to maintain a weight loss program if they can recognize physical changes and track their progress in tiny increments.

Using a BMI calculator, people can also monitor their body mass index (BMI).

3. Take part in regular exercise and physical activity

Weight loss can be aided by regular physical activity.
Exercise regularly is essential for both mental and physical health. For weight loss to be successful, increasing physical activity frequency in a deliberate and controlled manner is frequently essential.

It's best to engage in one hour of moderate-intensity exercise every day, like brisk walking. The Mayo Clinic advises that if an hour a day is not feasible, one should try to get at least 150 minutes per week.

Individuals who do not typically engage in physical activity should progressively increase both the quantity and intensity of their exercise. The best way to guarantee that regular exercise becomes a part of their routine is to take this strategy.

People may benefit psychologically by tracking their physical activity in the same way that maintaining a food journal can aid in weight loss. After logging food consumption and exercise, a person can use one of the many free mobile applications available to track their calorie balance.

If someone is new to exercising and finds the idea of a full workout frightening, they might start by practicing the following exercises to get more exercise:

Ascending the stairs
Dancing, playing outdoor games, raking leaves, walking dogs, gardening, and parking further away from a building entrance
It is unlikely that those with a low risk of coronary heart disease will need to be evaluated medically before beginning an exercise program.

However, for some individuals, particularly those who have diabetes, a previous medical evaluation may be advised. Anyone with questions concerning appropriate exercise dosages ought to consult a medical expert.

4. Get rid of liquid calories
Drinking tea, juice, soda with added sugar, or alcohol can result in the consumption of hundreds of calories every day. These are referred to as "empty calories" since they add extra energy content without improving nutrition.

A person should try to limit their intake to water, unsweetened tea, and coffee unless they are using smoothies as a meal substitute. A squeeze of fresh orange or lemon can add taste to water.

Do not confuse thirst with hunger. A glass of water can frequently quench one's hunger between meals that are scheduled.

5. Track quantities and measure servings
Gaining weight can occur by eating too much of any meal, including veggies that are low in calories.

As a result, consumers ought to refrain from consuming food straight out of the package or gauging the portion size. Serving size guidelines and measuring cups work well. Making assumptions increases the risk of overeating and consuming more food than is necessary.

When dining out, the size comparisons below can help keep an eye on how much food is consumed:

A golf ball is a quarter of a cup.
A half-cup is equivalent to a tennis ball.
A baseball is one cup.
A loose handful of nuts equals one ounce (oz).
One teaspoon is equivalent to one playing die.
A thumb tip is one tablespoon.
A deck of cards is three ounces of meat.
A single slice is a DVD.
These measurements are not precise, but when the right instruments are not available, they can assist someone in controlling how much food they eat.

6. Consume food attentively
A lot of people gain from mindful eating, which is paying close attention to what, when, how, where, and why they consume.

Being more aware of one's body leads directly to making healthier dietary choices.

In addition to trying to eat more slowly and savor their food, attentive eaters focus on the flavor. Giving a meal 20 minutes to complete allows the body to register all of the satiety cues.

After a meal, it's crucial to concentrate on feeling content rather than full and to keep in mind that not all "all-natural" or low-fat foods are necessarily healthy options.

In addition, people may think about the following queries before selecting a meal:

Is the "value" for the price in calories good?
Will it make you feel full?
Are the ingredients wholesome?
How much fat and sodium is in it, if it has a label?

7. Control Of Stimuli And Cues

Numerous environmental and social stimuli may promote overindulgent eating. For instance, some people are more prone to overindulge in food when they watch TV. Some find it difficult to hand over a dish of candies to another person without nibbling themselves.

People can come up with ways to modify their routine to limit these triggers by being conscious of what could make them want to nibble on empty calories.

8. Make A Plan In Advance

You'll lose more weight if you stock your kitchen with items that are low in calories and make organized meal plans.

Those who want to lose weight or maintain it should purge processed and junk food from their kitchen and make sure they always have the components needed to prepare quick and wholesome meals. By doing this, thoughtless, hurried, and unplanned eating can be avoided.

Making meal plans in advance of attending social gatherings or dining establishments may also facilitate the process.

9. Look For Social Assistance
Maintaining motivation is greatly enhanced by social support.
Accepting the help of those you love is essential to a successful weight loss program.

While some would choose to utilize social media to share their progress, others would want to ask friends or family to join them.

Additional resources for assistance could be:
A supportive social network group, individual therapy sessions, fitness clubs, or employee support initiatives at work

10. Remain Upbeat
Losing weight is a gradual process, so if the pounds do not come off as quickly as one had hoped, one may become disheartened.

Adhering to a weight reduction or maintenance program will involve some days that are more difficult than others. For a weight-loss program to be successful, the participant must stick with it and not give up when making changes to their behavior appears too hard.

It may be necessary for some people to reset their objectives, either by modifying their exercise regimen or the overall number of calories they intend to consume.

Maintaining A Positive Mindset And Perseveringly Attempting To Overcome Obstacles To Effective Weight Loss Is Crucial.

People can lose weight successfully without adhering to a diet regimen like Atkins or Slimming World. Rather, the emphasis should be on consuming fewer calories and increasing physical activity to attain an energy imbalance.

Reducing the overall amount of calories consumed is what leads to weight loss, not changing the ratios of protein, fat, and carbohydrates in the diet.

A 5- to 10-percent reduction in body weight over 6 months is an acceptable weight loss target to begin experiencing health advantages.

The majority of people may reach this target by cutting their daily caloric intake to between 1,600 and 1,000 calories.

Less than 1,000 calories a day won't give you enough nutrition for the entire day.

People prefer to consume less energy at a lower body weight, therefore after six months of dieting, the rate of weight loss normally decreases and body weight tends to stagnate. Regaining lost weight can be prevented by adhering to a weight maintenance program that includes regular exercise and healthy eating habits.

Prescription weight-loss drugs may be beneficial for those with a BMI of 30 or above who do not have any health issues connected to obesity. These may also be appropriate for patients with obesity-related conditions whose BMI is equal to or more than 27.

Medication should only be used in conjunction with the aforementioned lifestyle changes, though. Surgical therapy is a possibility if weight loss efforts fail and a person's BMI is 40 or higher.

In summary, sustaining weight loss necessitates a dedication to a healthy lifestyle with no time off. While people shouldn't feel bad about indulging in a special dinner out, celebrating a birthday, or having a festive holiday feast, they should also make an effort to stick to a diet that promotes healthful eating and regular exercise.

Those who do can experience concentration problems. It's simpler to gain back weight than to lose it.

When people make long-term lifestyle adjustments, they can lose weight and keep it off.

People who pay attention to what and how they eat, exercise regularly, and participate in daily physical activity will be effective in losing and maintaining their weight loss, regardless of any particular weight loss methods.

Keeping A Notepad With Your Diet And Exercise Schedule

Do you have a goal to live a healthy lifestyle? As you go through this journey, keeping a food journal or an activity log might be beneficial! You can identify issues, evaluate your progress, and become more conscious of your decisions by monitoring your health-related behaviors. Your Rocketbook notepad can assist, as usual!

Why It's Worth Keeping a Food Journal

If you're resolving to eat healthier in the new year, maintaining a food journal will be quite beneficial! You can identify the little indulgences that add up by keeping a food journal. Consuming a Coke here and a piece of candy there will quickly add up to a significant caloric intake. You can find a better substitute for those little, high-calorie goodies by keeping a meal journal.

Keeping a food journal might also assist you in identifying problematic trends. If you find that you always eat mindlessly at night to decompress from the day's stress, consider more constructive outlets such as exercise or meditation. Consider implementing Intermittent Fasting to rearrange your eating habits.

Food intolerances can also be found with the help of food logs. You should consider cutting out particular foods, such as dairy or gluten, from your diet if you feel bloated or ill in your stomach after eating them. At the very least, wait 30 minutes after eating before riding any spacecraft rides.

How to Keep a Food Journal in a Rocketbook Notepad

A meal journal is ideal to keep in a Rocketbook notebook! The executive size is particularly practical for tucking into a work bag or purse. It will always be with you when you need it.

Choose a page to keep a daily eating journal, with sections for breakfast, lunch, supper, snacks, and sweets or alcohol.
Choose a symbol for a food log folder in your preferred cloud location within the Rocketbook app. Upload the log and clean the slate at the end of each day. You'll accumulate an electronic food journal that you can review at a later time.

If you feel like you need more responsibility, you may show a friend your meal journal. Peer pressure from someone who periodically updates you on your progress can be sufficient to encourage you to make healthier decisions. Peer pressure works well in this situation.

Why It's Worth Keeping an Exercise Log?

Maintaining an exercise journal might assist you in reaching your fitness goals. You'll be responsible for your actions because the log is aware of your decisions to watch Netflix or work out (not that there's anything wrong with either). Furthermore, even though your large goal still seems a long way off, it can be motivating to track your progress over time when it comes to something as big as losing 25 pounds or finishing a marathon.

Another tool that helps with exercise decision-making is an exercise tracker. After you have a well-thought-out plan for the coming week, all that remains is to put it into action. You're more likely to persevere if you have fewer choices to make!

You'll eventually discover what comes naturally to you and what doesn't. Perhaps you find it difficult to work out in the evenings but excel at early workouts. You can gain a data-driven understanding of your issues and preferences by keeping an exercise record!

How to Keep an Exercise Log in a Rocketbook Notebook

Maintaining a weekly activity diary might be challenging; this is where an exercise log can help! An exercise log is an excellent tool for creating new movement-related habits, much like a food journal. Organize your workout record according to your individual tastes and movement objectives.

Finding Out How Much Exercise You Presently Get In

It's beneficial to assess your current level of activity before beginning a new workout regimen. This helps you create realistic goals and provides you with a baseline from which to develop. Here's a quick method to determine how active you are right now:

Maintain Track: Begin by recording all of the physical activities you engage in throughout a regular week in a journal or on your phone. This includes regular activities like walking the dog or cleaning the house, as well as structured routines like going to the gym or attending a yoga class.

Keep an Eye on Intensity: Take note of how intense each action is. Engaging in activities of a moderate level should cause your heart rate to increase somewhat and for you to perspire slightly. These might include gardening, cycling, or brisk strolling. Exercises that need more energy and force you to breathe more deeply include running, swimming, and sports.

Calculate the Estimated Time Spent by adding up the amount of time you spend exercising each day. Tell the truth and include everything, even if it's simply a quick circuit of the neighborhood. To find your total weekly activity time, multiply that by seven.

Compare to Recommendations: Review the adult physical activity guidelines that are advised. It is generally advised to engage in muscle-strengthening activities on two or more days per week in addition to 150 minutes of moderate-intensity aerobic activity or 75 minutes of vigorous-intensity aerobic activity per week.

Examine Your Lifestyle: Consider how your current amount of activity fits into your everyday routine. Are there chances to move more during the day, such as parking further away from the store or using the stairs rather than the elevator? Gradual adjustments might build up over time.

Examining how active you are right now will help you set more reasonable objectives and make significant adjustments to your routine. Recall that progress, not perfection, is the aim. Moving even a small amount contributes to a healthier, more active lifestyle.

CHAPTER 3: BUILDING A HARMONIOUS PLATE: TECHNIQUES FOR EATING WELL.

Finding a balance that suits you is the key to eating healthfully. Here are some useful advice to help you enjoy your meals and make healthy decisions:

Eat a Plate Full of Entire Foods: Stuff your plate full of entire, unprocessed foods such as fruits, vegetables, whole grains, lean meats, and healthy fats. These foods can help you feel full since they are high in nutrients.

Watch Your Portions: To prevent overindulging, be mindful of portion proportions. Though it's not necessary to measure everything, make an effort to pay attention to how much you consume. Sized dishes and bowls can assist you in controlling your serving sizes.

Plan: Set aside some time to organize your weekly menu for meals and snacks. This can assist you in making better decisions and preventing yourself from reaching for bad selections when you're hungry. To help you cope with hectic days, consider preparing certain meals ahead of time.

Savor Your Food: Take your time and enjoy your meals. When eating, try to focus on the tastes and textures of your meal rather than being distracted by TV or your phone. You may avoid overeating and increase your enjoyment of your food by eating attentively.

Maintain Your Hydration: Drink plenty of water throughout the day to stay hydrated. Make sure you're getting enough water in your diet because sometimes thirst might be confused with hunger. Try to get eight glasses a day at the very least, and more if the weather is hot or you're active.

Reduce Your Intake of Processed Foods: Processed foods are generally heavy in sugars, bad fats, and additives. Make an effort to reduce your intake of these items. Whenever feasible, choose whole foods instead. Your body will appreciate it!

Treat Yourself Occasionally: It's acceptable to occasionally treat yourself to your favorite foods. Feelings of limitation and resentment might result from total deprivation. Just watch how much you consume and indulge in sweets sparingly.

Listen to Your Body: Observe your feelings about various foods. You are free to skip anything if you disagree with it. Follow your body's instructions and eat when you're hungry until you're satisfied.

Seek Support: Encircle yourself with like-minded individuals in your family, friends, and online networks. When you're attempting to eat healthier, having someone to support you can help.

Be Kind to Yourself: Keep in mind that mistakes are inevitable and that nobody is flawless. Don't punish yourself for skipping a workout or eating poorly. You may always start over tomorrow since a new day awaits you.

You may create long-lasting healthy eating habits by implementing these easy techniques into your everyday routine. So let's toast to happy, healthier you and tasty, nourishing meals!

Creating A Menu That Offers A Variety Of Nutrient-dense Dishes

Creating a menu that includes a range of nutrient-dense meals is a great strategy to help your weight reduction efforts while making sure your body is getting the vital nutrients it needs. Here's a quick tip to help you put together a great and nutritious menu:

Embrace Variety: Begin by arranging your menu to feature a broad variety of dishes from various food groups. This guarantees that the nutrients and flavors in your meals are varied.

Lean Protein Sources: Include foods like poultry, turkey, fish, tofu, beans, lentils, and low-fat dairy products in your meals. Protein is crucial for weight loss since it keeps you feeling full and content.

Load Up on Fruits and Veggies: Include an abundance of vibrant fruits and vegetables to make them the focal point of your meals. To increase your consumption of vitamins, minerals, and fiber, try to fill half of your plate with fruits and vegetables.

Select Whole Grains: Refined grains should be avoided in favor of whole grains such as brown rice, quinoa, oats, barley, and whole wheat bread. Because whole grains have higher fiber and nutritional content, they help you feel fuller for longer and aid in weight loss.

Include Healthy Fats: Don't forget to include foods like avocados, nuts, seeds, olive oil, and fatty fish in your meals as sources of healthy fats. In addition to keeping you full between meals, healthy fats are essential for heart health.

Spice Things Up: Add complexity and dimension to your food without adding extra calories by adding herbs, spices, and other seasonings. Try a variety of taste combinations to keep your meals interesting and fulfilling.

Aim for Balance: Prepare well-balanced meals, containing a variety of healthy fats, carbohydrates, and protein. This equilibrium helps you avoid energy slumps during the day and maintain steady blood sugar levels.

Think About Dietary Needs: When organizing your menu, don't forget to account for any dietary requirements or preferences. There are lots of delectable selections to pick from, regardless of your dietary requirements—vegan, vegetarian, gluten-free, or otherwise.

Prepare Ahead of Time: Make meals and prepare in bulk to save time during the workweek. Invest some time on the weekend in meal preparation and preparing ingredients you can eat all week.

Be Creative: Don't be scared to experiment in the kitchen with different flavors and dishes. Seek guidance from cookbooks, internet recipes, or loved ones, and enjoy trying out various ingredients and cooking methods.

You may design a menu that is tasty and pleasurable to eat in addition to being nourishing and supporting your weight loss objectives if you keep these suggestions in mind. So, take out a pen and paper and begin organizing your meals for the upcoming week right now!

Learning The Proper Serving Sizes And How To Control Them.

Maintaining a balanced diet and successfully controlling your weight depends on knowing the appropriate portion sizes. The following basic advice will help you understand serving sizes and how to adjust them:

Examine Food Labels: Pay attention to the portion size that is specified on food labels. This makes it easier for you to calculate how many servings there are in a package and how much you're eating.

Employ Visual clues: To estimate portion sizes when labels aren't available, use visual clues. A portion of meat, for instance, should be approximately the size of your palm, whereas a portion of grains should be about the size of your fist.

Measure Portions: To precisely determine serving sizes, use a kitchen scale, measuring cups, and spoons. Although it may seem laborious at first, it teaches you what constitutes a proper portion.

Eating mindfully involves being aware of your body's signals of hunger and fullness. Eat more slowly, savor your food, and quit when you're full rather than full and bloated.

Eat at Your Own Risk: Restaurant portions are frequently enormous. To reserve half for later, think about sharing a dish with a buddy or immediately requesting a takeout container.

Load Up on Fruits and Veggies: Arrange fruits and vegetables to cover half of your plate. They help you feel full without consuming too many calories because they are high in nutrients but low in calories.

Watch Out for Hidden Calories: Avoid excessive portions of high-calorie meals and beverages, such as sugary snacks and sodas.

Use Smaller Bowls and Plates: Although it may seem counterintuitive, utilizing smaller dishes might deceive your mind into thinking you can eat less.

Plan Ahead: To prevent mindless nibbling, arrange your meals and snacks ahead of time. You may also portion up your snacks.

Seek Support: If you need advice or encouragement, don't be afraid to get in touch with friends, family, or a nutritionist. When it comes to your journey toward healthier eating habits, having someone to lean on can make all the difference.

By observing portion sizes and putting these easy-to-follow strategies into practice, you can control your weight, make better decisions, and feel more in charge of your eating routine.

Increasing The Amount Of Fruits, Vegetables, Lean Meats, And Whole Grains You Eat

Increasing the amount of whole grains, lean meats, fruits, and vegetables you eat is a fantastic approach to begin eating better. The following straightforward advice will assist you in including more of these wholesome items in your meals:

Whole Grains: Use whole grains, such as quinoa, brown rice, oats, and whole wheat bread, instead of processed grains. These choices will keep you feeling full and content longer since they include more fiber and nutrients.

Lean Meats: Opt for lean protein sources including fish, tofu, lentils, and legumes as well as skinless chicken. When compared to fatty portions of meat, they have less harmful fats and are higher in protein and other important nutrients.

Fruits: Make fruits your preferred dessert or snack. A range of fresh fruits can be kept on hand for simple and quick snacking, or they can be added to salads, smoothies, and yogurt for a touch of sweetness.

Veggies: At every meal, put colorful veggies on half of your plate. To obtain a range of vitamins and minerals, try to incorporate a variety of vegetables in your diet, whether it's through a crisp salad, roasted vegetables, or steaming greens.

Mix It Up: To make your meals interesting and delectable, try experimenting with different grains, meats, fruits, and vegetables. To keep things interesting in the kitchen, experiment with different ingredients and recipes.

Lean Cuts: When purchasing meat, choose lean varieties such as turkey, chicken breast, or lean beef, or hog cuts. Before cooking, trim off any apparent fat to maintain a lean, nutritious dinner.

Snack Wisely: Go for whole foods instead of processed snacks, such as a handful of nuts and seeds, fresh fruit, or raw vegetables with hummus. These choices are tasty, filling, and nutritious all at once.

Include Veggies Everywhere: Try to include as many vegetables as you can in your meals. Top sandwiches and wraps with extra vegetables, incorporate shredded carrots or zucchini into meatballs or burgers or add spinach or peppers to omelets.

Plan: Set aside some time to organize your weekly menu for meals and snacks. To ensure you have wholesome options available at all times, stock up on whole grains, lean proteins, fruits, and vegetables.

Savor the Procedure: Above all, enjoy yourself while doing it! Try out different flavors and ingredients; don't worry about getting every dish just right. Concentrate on implementing tiny, enduring adjustments that you find enjoyable and fulfilling.

You may promote your general health and well-being and provide your body with important nutrients by increasing the amount of fruits, vegetables, whole grains, and lean meats in your diet.

CHAPTER 4: PRACTICAL GUIDANCE FOR A WELL-BEING DIET

Prepare Meals In Advance To Save Time And Select Healthier Options.

Arrange Your Meals: Making a weekly meal plan guarantees that you're eating a balanced, nutrient-dense diet by providing you with a clear outline of what to eat. Spend some time each day deciding what you will eat for snacks, dinner, lunch, and morning. Take into account your diet, timetable, and any ingredients you already have on hand. By being proactive, you can steer clear of impulsive purchases and last-minute decisions, which can eventually help you make healthier food choices.

After you've scheduled your meals, it's time to go shopping and get all the ingredients you'll need. Making a list before you go to the grocery shop keeps you organized and helps you remember what you need. Before creating your list, go through your pantry, refrigerator, and freezer to make sure you don't buy duplicates of anything you already own. To make your shopping trip more productive, divide your list into categories such as vegetables, dairy, and pantry necessities.

Set Aside Time for Meal Preparation: Set aside a set amount of time per week for meal preparation. This could take a couple of hours on a Sunday afternoon, or on a day that suits your schedule the most. Meal preparation should be prioritized and treated like an appointment, just like any other significant work. You'll be more likely to follow through and maintain your healthy eating goals if you set aside time for meal planning.

Ingredients for Batch Cooking: Batch cooking is the process of preparing a large number of ingredients at once so they can be used in several meals over the week. For instance, you can prepare a large quantity of brown rice, quinoa, or grilled chicken breasts to use as the base for other recipes. By reducing the amount of cooking you have to do on hectic weeknights, batch cooking guarantees that you always have wholesome options available and saves time.

Utilize Containers with Portion Control: Storage of your prepared meals and snacks can be done conveniently with portion-controlled containers. It's simple to divide out food and regulate serving quantities using these containers because they have different sections and sizes. By utilizing portion-controlled containers, you can avoid overindulging and make sure that every meal contains the proper ratio of nutrients. They're also perfect for eating on the go because you can just take a container and go.

Label and Organize: Make sure to label your prepared meals with the dish's name and the day it was made. This guarantees that you're eating meals when they're still fresh and helps you keep track of what's in your refrigerator. Make sure your meals are readily accessible by arranging them in the refrigerator or freezer. To make your lunchtime routine more efficient, think about organizing goods by meal type or putting comparable items together.

Provide a Range of Options: When it comes to meal preparation, variety is essential. When preparing meals, try to incorporate a variety of items such as grains, veggies, proteins, and sauces. This guarantees that you're getting a variety of nutrients in your diet in addition to keeping things interesting. To keep your taste buds engaged, don't be scared to try new ingredients and dishes.

Remember to Include Snacks: A meal planning regimen should include snacks. Making healthful snacks in advance can help stop mindless snacking on less wholesome options. For easy and quick snacks, chop fruits and vegetables, divide out nuts and seeds, or make your own energy bars or trail mix. Keeping wholesome snacks on hand facilitates the process of avoiding temptation and maintaining your fitness regimen.

Maintain Flexibility: Although meal planning will assist you in adhering to your healthy eating objectives, it's crucial to maintain flexibility and adaptability. Plans can change as life happens. Don't be afraid to switch things up and replace meals as needed if you find yourself with unexpected leftovers or you're not in the mood for a particular one. Make thoughtful decisions that promote your general well-being while paying attention to your body and honoring your cravings.

Savor the Benefits: There are many advantages to meal planning, including time savings and improved health. You'll save time during the week and lessen the stress of having to decide what to eat if you make the effort to plan and prepare your meals in advance. You'll also have better access to healthier selections, which will make it simpler for you to follow your diet plan and feed your body nourishing foods. Accept meal preparation as an opportunity to prioritize your health and well-being and to take care of yourself.

Rotate Your Menu: Changing up your menu regularly will keep things interesting and new. This keeps mealtimes interesting and guarantees that you're consuming a diverse range of nutrients from various foods. To broaden your cooking skills, try experimenting with new dishes and incorporating seasonal food.

Make Smoothie Packs: If you're looking for a healthy and fast breakfast or snack option, make smoothie packs in advance. Put your preferred fruits, leafy greens, and protein sources in separate freezer bags. When you're ready to eat, just combine it with a drink. By doing this, you guarantee that you begin your day with a nutritious dose of vitamins and minerals while also saving time in the morning.

Make Use of Multi-Functional Appliances: If you're looking to streamline your meal prep process, consider using an air fryer, pressure cooker, or slow cooker. These multipurpose kitchen appliances enable you to cook a variety of foods, from soups and stews to roasted vegetables and protein-rich meals, in big quantities with little effort.

Practice Food Safety: To avoid contracting a foodborne illness, use the correct food safety procedures when preparing meals. Before and after usage, give all surfaces, utensils, and containers a thorough cleaning and sanitization. Reheat leftovers to the right temperature before consuming them, and store perishable goods in the freezer or refrigerator as soon as possible. Additionally, when preparing meals, keep raw and cooked items apart to prevent cross-contamination.

Snack Packs for Batch Preparation: Divide up wholesome snacks into discrete bags or containers for convenient grab-and-go options all week long. Incorporate a blend of fiber, protein, and good fats to help you feel full in between meals. Trail mix with nuts, seeds, and dried fruit is one example, as is cheese and whole grain crackers, or Greek yogurt and fruit.

mark Cooking directions: To make reheating easier, mark containers with cooking directions when batch-preparing meals or ingredients. To guarantee that your dishes are reheated safely and retain their quality and flavor, include recommended cooking times and procedures. This removes uncertainty and facilitates easy and speedy food preparation.

Play around with Flavor Boosters: Try different herbs, spices, sauces, and marinades to enhance the flavor of your food. These flavor enhancers give your food more depth and complexity without using a lot of sugar, salt, or unhealthy fats. To keep your taste buds happy, get creative in the kitchen, and don't be afraid to explore new flavor combinations.

Make a Plan for Leftovers: Seize the chance to cut down on food waste and save time by embracing leftovers. Make sure to plan and make extra food so that you have leftovers for other meals. To maintain freshness, store leftovers in portion-controlled containers and mark them with the date. To keep things interesting, you can use leftovers to make new meals or enjoy them just the way they are.

Remain Hydrated: Drink plenty of water throughout the day, particularly when preparing meals. To stay hydrated, always have a water bottle on hand and take frequent breaks to sip on water. In addition to promoting general health, enough hydration helps reduce headaches, weariness, and food cravings during meal preparation.

Practice Mindful Eating: Lastly, during the week and when preparing meals, engage in mindful eating. Savor each bite of your food, taking the time to appreciate its flavors, textures, and colors. Eat mindfully of your body's signals of hunger and fullness, and take your time to enjoy your food. Emotional and excessive eating can be avoided by practicing mindful eating, which also fosters a positive relationship with food.

Choosing Filling Snacks That Won't Hinder Your Attempts To Lose Weight.

Selecting foods that satisfy your hunger without impeding your weight loss efforts is essential when it comes to snacking when trying to lose weight. Here's how to pick snacks that won't undermine your attempts to lose weight:

Nutrient-Packed Snacks: Choose snacks that are high in nutrients but low in calories. Consider lean proteins, nuts, seeds, crisp vegetables, and fresh fruits. These foods give you the fiber, vitamins, and minerals you need to feel full without gaining weight.

Make protein a priority. When it comes to feeling full and content in between meals, protein is your buddy. Nuts, cottage cheese, Greek yogurt, and hard-boiled eggs are all excellent snack options. They prevent hunger and support the maintenance of muscular mass when losing weight.

Fiber-Rich Snacks: Adding fiber to your snacks helps them feel fuller for longer. Choose high-fiber snacks such as whole grains, legumes, fruits, and veggies. These foods help regulate weight, promote digestive health, and reduce cravings.

Low-Calorie Snacks: Choose foods that are high in volume and nutrients while being reasonably priced. A bowl of broth-based soup, air-popped popcorn, or raw vegetables with hummus are low-calorie options that satisfy your hunger without piling on the pounds.

Portion control is important since, if you're not careful, even nutritious snacks can cause overeating. Plan your snack portions to prevent mindless snacking. To assist you in staying on track with your objectives, stick to single servings or pre-portioned containers.

Avoid Processed Foods: Snacks that have been through a lot of processing are frequently high in added sugars, bad fats, and empty calories. Choose whole, less processed meals instead of chips, cookies, and candy bars. Your body will be grateful for the nutrition and continuous vitality.

Drink plenty of water since sometimes hunger might pass for thirst. To stay hydrated, make sure you're consuming plenty of water throughout the day. Avoiding thirst can help you control your desires and avoid mindless snacking.

Plan Ahead: Being prepared will help you resist temptation when hunger strikes. Keep a supply of healthful snacks on hand so you can grab them quickly when hunger strikes. Making your snacks in advance guarantees that you always have wholesome options available and lessens the chance that you'll grab junk food.

Pay heed to your body's signals of hunger and fullness by listening to them. Select munchies that will satiate your appetite without making you feel full or lethargic. Overeating can be avoided and your weight reduction journey can be supported by eating thoughtfully and paying attention to your body's cues.

When you snack, try to eat mindfully by paying attention to the flavors and textures of the food. Enjoy the tastes, textures, and fragrances of your snack slowly. You can avoid overeating and feel more pleased with lesser servings when you eat attentively.

Satiating Fats: To boost sensations of fullness and satiety, include healthy fats in your snacks. Select unsaturated fat-containing foods like avocado, olives, nuts, and seeds. Essential fatty acids included in these meals promote general health and may help reduce cravings.

Balance Macros: To keep you feeling full and energized, choose snacks that have a good ratio of fats, proteins, and carbohydrates. For instance, eat whole grain crackers with cheese or apple slices with almond butter. By balancing macros, blood sugar crashes and spikes can be avoided and a continuous release of energy can be guaranteed.

Pre-portioned snacks: If you're a sugar addict, these snacks can help you sate your cravings without going overboard. Go for tiny servings of dried fruit, dark chocolate, or homemade energy balls that are packed with healthy components like dates, almonds, and oats.

Snacks that are High in Water Content: Snacks high in water content might help you stay hydrated and full. Pick for pleasant fruit and vegetable smoothies, cucumber slices, or cubed watermelon as hydrated options. Dehydration-induced hunger cues can also be avoided by maintaining water.

Snack Combos: To maintain interest and satisfaction, experiment with different snack combos. Combine several food groups to make tasty and well-balanced snacks. For instance, have a little dish of healthy grain crackers with tuna salad or sliced turkey with cucumber and hummus.

Whole Food Selections: Whenever feasible, use minimally processed, whole foods for your snacking. These nutrient-dense meals offer long-lasting energy without the additional sugars and harmful ingredients of processed snacks. For a filling snack, go for items like raw almonds, baby carrots, or a portion of whole fruit.

Customize to Taste: Adjust your snack selections based on your dietary requirements and personal tastes. Try a variety of flavors, textures, and ingredient combinations until you find ones that you like. There are many delectable and healthful snack options to try, regardless of your preference for sweet, savory, or a mix of the two.

Snacks After Exercise: If you exercise, select foods that will aid in your recuperation and provide energy for your muscles. Choose a snack that includes protein for muscle repair and carbohydrates for energy replacement after working out. A protein smoothie, a banana with peanut butter, or Greek yogurt with berries are all great post-workout options.

Social Support: Be in the company of loved ones who encourage and support your efforts to improve your health and well-being. Encourage one another to choose wholesome snacks by sharing your snack selections with others. On your weight loss journey, having a supportive network may keep you accountable and motivated.

Appreciate Your Progress: Acknowledge your accomplishments along the route, such as the wise snacks you chose. Celebrate the little successes and accomplishments you have along the way to losing weight. Whether it's overcoming temptation, attempting a novel, healthful food, or accomplishing a little goal, celebrate your successes and use them as inspiration to carry on.

You may maintain your weight loss objectives while satisfying your cravings by selecting foods that are nourishing and filling. Try out a few different combinations to see which one suits you the best, then reap the rewards of long-lasting energy and fullness all day.

Using Mindful Eating Techniques To Eat Less And Appreciate Your Food More.

Do you have the experience of being so hungry that you eat almost without tasting it? Done that, been there. However, what if I told you there was a way to enjoy your food more, eat less without feeling deprived, and slow down? Let us introduce mindful eating.

Imagine yourself enjoying a delicious lunch, but instead of going straight for the food, you pause to enjoy the flavors, textures, and colors on your plate. Chewing gently and truly tasting the flavors, you relish every bite. Eating with awareness feeds not only your physical needs but also your spiritual well-being.

Being able to recognize your body's signals of hunger and fullness is one of the best things about mindful eating. Rather than idly scarfing down a bag of chips, you begin to notice how your body is feeling. Are you eating only out of boredom or habit, or are you truly hungry? You can learn to eat when you're hungry and stop eating when you're full, even if there is food left on your plate, by learning to listen to your body.

Let's also discuss portion management. You can learn to listen to your body's natural cues about when to stop eating by practicing mindful eating. Say goodbye to the days of mindlessly overindulging in food and then feeling full hours later. You may enjoy your meals without going overboard if you serve yourself smaller servings and take the time to truly enjoy every bite.

However, eating mindfully involves more than just what you put in your mouth. Distractions like TV and phones should be avoided during dining so that you may concentrate entirely on the meal. You'll be astounded at how much more fulfilling eating is when you're not dozing off or multitasking.

The best part is that mindful eating doesn't require you to abide by rigid guidelines or give up meals you enjoy. It's about approaching food with thankfulness, inquiry, and compassion. So feel free to indulge in that spaghetti dish or piece of cake. Just take your time and enjoy every mouthwatering taste.

Imagine that when you're eating, you pause for a moment rather than cramming food into your mouth while aimlessly browsing through your phone. Your mouth starts to wet with anticipation as you inhale the food's aroma. As you bite into something, you allow the flavors and textures to truly sing on your tongue. This is what mindful eating is all about.

But the story doesn't end with the dinner; it begins long before you reach for a fork. A conscious mind starts with aware eating. Before you eat, take time to check in with yourself. Do you eat because you're bored, acting on an emotion, or are you genuinely hungry? Understanding your body's demands and making more deliberate decisions about what and when to eat are made possible by being aware of your hunger cues.

Let's now discuss distractions. How frequently do you eat while watching TV or using the web, hardly noticing what's on your plate? When we have conflicting priorities, it is simple to succumb to the temptation of mindless eating. However, you can completely participate in the eating experience when you block out all other distractions and concentrate just on your meal. Smaller quantities will satisfy you more, you'll appreciate your food more, and you'll notice flavors more strongly.

Another important component of mindful eating is portion control. Pay attention to your body's internal cues rather than depending on outside indications such as portion sizes or plate sizes. Even if there is food remaining on your plate, pay attention to how your body feels as you eat and quit when you're satisfied. Paying attention to your body's natural signals of hunger and fullness will help you stay within a healthy weight range and prevent overeating.

Not to be overlooked is thankfulness. Eating can be made more enjoyable and a stronger bond can be formed with food if you take a moment to be grateful for it, for the farmers who raised it, the hands that prepared it, or the planet that gave it. Meals are more likely to be savored and healthier decisions are made when you approach them with appreciation and thankfulness.

Eating mindfully can be a game-changer in a world where we're always racing from one activity to the next. Thus, take it slowly, pay attention, and truly enjoy the food that's on your plate. Your taste senses and body will appreciate it.

CHAPTER 5: THE IMPORTANCE OF HYDRATION

Acknowledging The Advantages Of Drinking More Water To Lose Weight.

When it comes to weight loss, realizing the advantages of increasing your water intake might make all the difference. Here's how drinking more water can truly help:

Manage Your Hunger: Have you ever noticed that occasionally, you're not hungry—just thirsty? You can reduce your appetite and feel less hungry by drinking water before meals.

Boost Metabolism: Hydration helps to maintain a healthy metabolism. Your body can burn calories more effectively when you're well-hydrated, which is essential for losing weight.

Calorie-Free Hydration: Water has no calories, in contrast to sugary beverages. You can reduce your total caloric intake without even trying you replace those high-calorie drinks with water.

Improved Workouts: Hydration is essential for achieving maximum efficiency when exercising. Your energy and endurance levels increase when you're well-hydrated, which makes it simpler to crush your exercises and burn more calories.

Promotes Fat Loss: Your body can't metabolize fat as effectively when you're thirsty. By ensuring that your body's fat-burning mechanisms are operating at maximum efficiency, drinking enough water can help you lose weight more quickly.

Reduces Bloating: Even though it may seem paradoxical, increasing your water intake can assist lessen bloating. Your body is less prone to retain extra water weight when you're well hydrated, which makes you feel lighter and less puffy.

Aids Digestion: To maintain a healthy digestive system, you must drink plenty of water. It aids in the breakdown of meals, nutritional absorption, and prevention of bloating and constipation, all of which can undermine your attempts to lose weight.

Maintains Energy Levels: Being dehydrated can make you feel exhausted and lethargic, which makes it more difficult to remain active and driven. You can make sure you have the energy you need to go through your day and your workouts by making sure you drink enough water.

Reduces Liquid Calorie Intake: Sugar-filled beverages such as juice and soda can easily pack on the extra calories. Instead, go for water to reduce your calorie consumption without compromising your hydration.

Benefits to Your General Health: Drinking enough water is important for your general health as well as for helping you lose weight. Drink plenty of water to maintain a healthy body, as it aids in temperature regulation and toxin removal.

That means the next time you're feeling peckish or lethargic, pick up a glass of water. It may be exactly what your body needs to continue making progress toward your weight loss objectives.

Tips For Staying Hydrated During The Day: Drink Responsibly, And Avoid Overindulging In Sugary Beverages.

Being aware of what and how much you drink is crucial to ensuring that you stay hydrated throughout the day. Here are some easy tips to help you maintain adequate hydration:

Water is Your Best Friend: H2O is the most effective way to stay hydrated. Carry a water bottle with you at all times, and drink from it frequently.

Establish Self-Reminders: It's simple to forget to drink water when life gets hectic. To remind yourself to take a sip, try using your phone's reminder feature or placing sticky notes everywhere.

Mix it Up: If you're not a fan of plain water, consider flavoring it. For a cool twist, add some slices of cucumber or lemon to your water.

Eat Water: It may surprise you to learn that some foods can also help you stay hydrated. Eat veggies like cucumber and celery as a snack, or nibble on fruits high in water content like watermelon, oranges, or grapes.

Limit Your Consumption of Sugary Drinks: Although they may taste nice, sugary drinks like juice and soda aren't the greatest option for staying hydrated. In the long term, they may make you feel more thirsty. When feasible, stick to water or other unsweetened beverages.

Pay Attention to Your Urine: Although it may sound disgusting, your urine can reveal a lot about how hydrated you are. Urine should ideally be a pale yellow color; if it's darker, you should drink more water.

Avoid Being Thirsty: Avoid reaching for a drink when you're already feeling thirsty. You're already close to becoming dehydrated by the time you experience thirst. Drink water frequently during the day to avoid being thirsty.

Hydrate Before and After Exercise: Drink lots of water before, during, and after your workout to avoid being dehydrated and sweaty.

Moderate Your Alcohol Consumption: Drinking alcohol can cause dehydration, so if you do enjoy a few drinks, make sure you balance them out with lots of water.

In the end, paying attention to your body's needs is the greatest method to maintain proper hydration. When you're thirsty, sip water and pay attention to how you're feeling. That's all there is to it!

Maintain Water Accessible: Keep a filled water bottle in your car, on your desk, or in your bag to make it simple to get to water. Water that is easily accessible increases the likelihood that you will frequently drink it.

Establish Hydration Objectives: Assign yourself daily hydration objectives, such as consuming a specific amount of glasses or liters of water during the day. Setting a goal for yourself can keep your hydration efforts on track.

Use a Straw: Using a straw can make it easier for some people to consume more water. For added convenience and enjoyment, try pairing your water bottle with a reusable straw.

Hydrate First Thing in the Morning: Upon waking up, sip a glass of water to kick-start your day. This helps your body replenish fluids after a restful night and revs up your metabolism for the coming day.

Monitor Your Intake: Use a pen and paper notebook or a water tracking app to keep track of how much water you consume each day. You may be inspired to drink more and meet your hydration objectives if you can observe your progress.

Choose meals High in Water: Apart from fruits and vegetables, include meals high in water in your diet, like smoothies, yogurt, and soups. These items can help you stay hydrated by adding to your overall fluid intake.

Hydrate Before Meals: Have a glass of water before every meal to help hydrate your body and manage portion amounts to avoid overindulging.

Make it a Habit: Develop the habit of drinking enough water throughout the day. For example, have a glass of water when you wake up before you eat, and right before bed.

Pay Attention to Your Thirst: Your body will tell you when you're thirsty and should increase your water intake. When you notice these cues, take action by sipping water whenever you feel thirsty.

Be Patient: Keep in mind that improving your hydration habits takes time, so it's acceptable to start small. Be kind to yourself and acknowledge your accomplishments as you go.

CHAPTER 6: KNOWLEDGE OF CALORIES: HOW MUCH IS SUFFICIENT?

Learning About The Principles And Methods Of Calorie Counting.

Anyone looking to gain or reduce weight safely may find that counting calories is helpful. But it's also critical to consume calories from wholesome foods, obtain the recommended amount of sleep and exercise, and manage stress levels.

Although it may seem difficult to count calories, there are several resources available, such as online calculators and applications.

A unit of measurement is calorie. They provide a means of expressing energy levels.

People seem to be most familiar with Reliable Source with "big" calories, which indicate how much energy a food or beverage contains.

Why are calories important?

Energy from calories is essential for maintaining life and health. It supports vital biological processes, including cell functionTrusted Source.

For example, the body turns food's calories into energy. Depending on its immediate demands, it either uses this energy right away or stores it for later.

For what reason do you count them?

Calorie counting has numerous benefits. In general, this enables an individual to calculate the amount of energy they use each day.

A person usually starts to acquire weight if they consume more calories than their body expels. A person usually begins to lose weight if they consume less than what their body needs.

A person is at risk if, over an extended period, foods high in simple sugars serve as their main source of excess calories. Reliable Source of:

Anxiety and depression.
Apnea during sleep.
Osteoarthritis, gallstones, gallbladder disease, and issues with fertility.
Gout, type 2 diabetes, nonalcoholic fatty liver disease, and heart disease.
Hypertension stroke malignancies, including colon and breast cancer.
Individuals who are upping their activity levels dramatically require additional calories to balance out what they are burning.

An individual who consumes insufficient calories runs the risk of:
Rise of weight due to a reduction in cortisol production
Abnormalities in heartbeat
Deteriorating skeletal structure
The decrease in skeletal muscle, heart, and kidney mass
Urreversible organ damage
Heart arrest

What number does the body require?
The recommended daily intake of calories for an individual is determined by their:

Height, gender, age, and degree of activity.

An online tool from the National Institutes of Health (NIH)Trusted Source determines the number of calories an individual needs to consume to achieve their desired weight.

The calculator also accounts for how long the user wants to take to accomplish this aim.

The best applications for tracking calories
Calorie-counting applications for iPhone and Android are available for free, and they include:

MyFitnessPal, which offers free recipes and health articles in addition to tracking calories and macro- and micronutrients.

MyNetDiary, which monitors steps taken, water consumed, and calories consumed at each meal.

Lose It, which monitors body measurements, foods, sleep, water, daily exercise, and weight and body fat.

My Diet Diary, which includes forums for assistance and records calories, exercise, and hydration.

How to measure and weigh servings
Portion sizes are typically indicated on food and drink labels in the form of cups, ounces, grams, pieces, slices, or numerals.

Taking quantities into account might assist trusted Sources in keeping a healthy weight and calorie counting.

For instance, an individual can measure out a portion of 2/3 cup of ice cream, as indicated on the label, to determine precisely how many calories they are ingesting. However, the individual would only need to take 1/3 cup to stay on track if they only had 115 calories remaining in their daily allotment.

Having a precise set of cups, scales, and other measuring tools close at hand is beneficial.

A well-rounded diet
When establishing weight or fitness objectives, consuming more or less calories should never be the only factor taken into account. Maintaining a healthy weight is influenced by stress, sleep, and activity levels.

Furthermore, the type and quality of food or drink consumed can have a big impact on the source of calories.

Though the same number of calories from various foods can have varied impacts, all calories are converted to energy.

For instance, consuming the recommended daily amount of calories from foods high in refined carbs and added sugar will boost blood sugar levels, which in turn increases the amount of fat stored in the body.

In a similar vein, consuming a lot of calories from meals high in animal fats—especially red meat—may raise your risk of developing some malignancies, such as esophageal cancer.

It is essential to receive your calories from a balanced diet rich in fruits, vegetables, whole grains, and healthy fats like olive oil, almonds, and avocados. The nutrients that the body requires to function are present in these foods.

A diet high in refined sugar may be especially problematic since it can cause insulin spikes, which cause fat cells to accumulate calories. The body reacts with hunger since these calories don't contain the essential nutrients.

Alcohol also contains a lot of these "empty" calories and can lead to inadvertent weight gain.

Some Advice On Calorie Counting

The following techniques could be useful while tracking calories:

Utilizing an app that counts calories to keep a food journal.
Utilizing a meal plan that is intended to supply the required amount of calories and strive for gradual, stable weight changes

Because counting calories entails keeping track of the amount of energy that is being absorbed by the body each day, it can help people achieve and maintain their fitness and weight objectives.

Numerous apps and web resources may calculate and track an individual's daily caloric requirements to meet their objectives.

It is imperative that people wishing to modify their weight also take into account their stress and physical activity levels, as well as the quantity and quality of their sleep. Each of these elements is important.

Determining The Optimal Balance Between Calories Burned And Consumed.

Maintaining your health and controlling your weight both depend on consuming and burning the same amount of calories. Here's how to locate the ideal location:

Know Your Body: To begin with, ascertain your basal metabolic rate (BMR), which is the amount of calories required for your body to function while at rest. To calculate your BMR based on variables like age, height, weight, and activity level, use one of the many online calculators available.

Factor in Activity: Take into account your daily activity level. Calorie-burning activities include walking, exercising, and household tasks. You will require more calories to feed your body the more active you are.

Calculate Your Sum: To find your total daily energy expenditure, add your body mass index (BMR) to the number of calories you burn from exercise. (TDEE). This is how many calories you must consume daily to stay at your present weight.

Establish Your Objectives: Modify your caloric intake based on your desired weight loss, maintenance, or growth. Try to eat less than your TDEE to lose weight. Adjust your consumption to your TDEE to maintain your weight. Eat more calories than your TDEE to gain mass.

Track Your Intake: Use a food journal or a smartphone app to keep track of what you're consuming. This keeps you responsible and ensures that you are not eating too much or too little.

Select Carefully: Make an effort to eat foods high in nutrients, which will both satiate your hunger and supply vital vitamins and minerals. Consider entire grains, fruits, veggies, lean meats, and healthy fats. These foods nourish your body in addition to keeping you full.

Pay Attention to Your Body: Observe your body's signals of hunger and fullness. Consume food only when you're hungry and quit when you're full. When it comes to how much fuel it requires, your body is the expert.

Have patience: Recall that it takes trial and error to find the ideal balance. If things don't go smoothly at first, don't give up. Remain adaptable and change course as necessary.

Seek Support: Don't be afraid to ask for assistance if you're having trouble maintaining your equilibrium. A qualified nutritionist or registered dietitian can offer you individualized advice and support to help you accomplish your objectives.

You can discover the right balance between calories burned and absorbed by your body by paying attention to what you eat and how active you are. This will help you maintain a healthy weight and way of life.

Avoid Common Mistakes That Could Make Your Weight Loss Efforts More Difficult.

Avoiding common blunders might help you lose weight and prevent you from reaching your goals. Here are a few things to watch out for:

Having unrealistic expectations: Losing weight quickly won't last and will just cause frustration and disappointment. Instead, strive for a consistent, progressive weight loss of one to two pounds every week.

Meal Skipping: Although skipping meals can seem like a simple approach to reduce calories, it can have the opposite effect by slowing down your metabolism and leading to overeating later in the day. To maintain steady energy levels, consume regular, well-balanced meals and snacks.

Relying on Fad Diets: Fad diets that promise rapid results sometimes include drastically reducing calorie intake or eliminating entire food groups, neither of which are long-term sustainable. Instead, concentrate on altering your eating habits in tiny, long-lasting ways.

Overestimating Exercise Calories: Although exercise is crucial for losing weight, it's simple to overestimate how many calories you burn when working out. Instead of using your workout as an excuse to overindulge in junk food, concentrate on building a balanced diet.

Ignoring Portion Sizes: Eating big portions of even healthful foods can lead to weight gain. To help you manage your portions, pay attention to portion sizes and make use of instruments like food scales or measuring cups.

Mindless Eating: Consuming food when preoccupied, like when watching TV or working at a desk, can cause overindulgence without the person even recognizing it. By paying attention to your food and enjoying every bite, you can practice mindful eating.

Consuming Fluid Calories: Sugar-filled beverages, alcoholic beverages, and calorically dense coffee drinks can rapidly accumulate and undermine your attempts to reduce weight. Instead, stick to black coffee, unsweetened tea, or water.

Not Getting Enough Sleep: Hormones that control appetite and hunger can be upset by not getting enough sleep, which can cause cravings and overeating. To help you reach your weight loss objectives, aim for 7 to 9 hours of good sleep per night.

Ignoring Emotional Eating: You can undermine your attempts to lose weight if you use food as a coping method for stress, boredom, or other emotions. Look for other ways to deal with your feelings, including working out, keeping a diary, or speaking with a friend.

Not Seeking Help: It can be difficult to attempt weight loss on your own. To keep yourself accountable and motivated, ask friends, family, or a support group for assistance.

You can position yourself for long-term success in accomplishing your weight loss objectives by staying away from these typical blunders and concentrating on wholesome, long-lasting practices.

CHAPTER 7: MOVING YOUR BODY: SELECTING ENJOYABLE EXERCISE

Trying Out Different Types Of Exercise To Determine What Works For You.

Eating a wholesome diet that permits a calorie deficit combined with the greatest exercise for weight loss is the key to healthily losing weight. It can indeed be challenging to lose weight without exercising, even though following the finest diets for weight reduction and developing general healthy habits will help you look and feel your best.

The best workouts to shed pounds

1. Sprinting

Sprinting is one of the greatest and easiest ways to burn calories, regardless of your feelings about the sport. You can do it without a treadmill. Simply put on your shoes and get out. The minutes and miles will fly by if you run in intervals, picking up and dropping your pace. Run in fartleks, which translates to "speed play" from Swedish, in which you accelerate past each other and slow down when you reach a hydrant or street lamp.

"Changing up your workouts is the best way to burn calories while running." If you're working out the same way every week, your body won't have anything to adjust to. Change up your workouts by varying your pace, adding short spurts of quicker jogging, and switching up the kinds of runs you perform. Variability is essential for ongoing adaptation, whether it be in the form of intervals, easy and difficult, or gradual and steady.

Running slow is comparatively easy on your body in terms of perceived exertion, but running fast at 80% of your capability is even tougher, pushing your body even further to its limitations. This is because sprinting helps activate the core and gives shorter durations of runs at higher intensities. Your body will become accustomed to this level of stress as a result. "The next time, instead of running on the road, go to a track or soccer field and do some sprints; there is something to be said about learning to be comfortable being uncomfortable on your runs."

2. Strolling

If you're not into running, think about strolling as a weight loss strategy. "One of the best exercises for weight loss is walking. This is a low-impact weight-bearing exercise. By adding weight vests, Nordic sticks, wrist or ankle weights, and climbing hills, one can vary the speed, duration, and intensity of this exercise, which boosts energy expenditure, strolling 30 minutes per day, most days of the week, at a moderate speed can assist with weight reduction endeavours.

Strolling is particularly beneficial for people who need low-impact exercise, are starting a weight loss program, and have diabetes because it can assist lower blood glucose levels. This is something that White emphasizes.

No matter what your fitness objectives are, walking every day has a lot of advantages. According to White, a few of these advantages could be assisting in the maintenance of a healthy weight, enhanced cardiovascular health, heightened mood and vigor, decreased stress, and enhanced balance and coordination.

3. Trekking

Both trekking and strolling are healthy ways to get exercise. Strolling, however, can be a better choice if you want to walk for more calories expended and to reap the benefits of weight loss. "To shed pounds, climbing will assist you with making the fundamental calorie deficiency more actually than strolling will." This is on the grounds that climbing is fairly more enthusiastically than level strolling.

This is because trekking is somewhat harder than level walking. Walking over the rougher terrain, hills, and altitudes will put more strain on your body but also help strengthen your legs and core, improve your balance, and burn more calories. "All things considered, hiking is a fantastic way to get outside, take in the scenery, and get some exercise."

4. Leap Rope

Want to make working out a little more enjoyable? Take a swing at a jump rope. "Jumping rope will help you build power while lowering your risk of injury and is a great way to burn calories, improve cardiovascular health, and tone your entire body."

For burning calories, jumping rope is on par with running, cycling, and swimming. About 12 calories would be burned every minute by an adult weighing 150 pounds leaping at what is considered an average pace. This is a pretty good burn, equal to the pace of an 8½-mile run. Additionally, there are a ton of advantages to jump ropes, such as:

Increases your heart rate
Uses a variety of muscle groups
Increases bone density
Attainable almost anyplace
Enhances coordination and balance

Try this Crossrope routine: Begin with 60 seconds of jump roping in a freestyle manner. One foot, two feet, alternate, skip, or twist your hips can all be used for jumping. This one can provide some entertainment. After that, lower your rope and perform mountain climbing for 30 seconds. Come back for a 60-second jump rope freestyle session. Finish with a 30-second plank. After two minutes of rest, repeat the cycle. Finish all three rounds.

5. Strength Exercises

You can increase your metabolism and gain lean muscle mass by engaging in strength exercises. Because your metabolism is higher when you have more muscle, you burn less fat overall. "More fat is lost and more calories are ignited with a better ability to burn calories."

Osteoporosis can also be avoided with resistance exercise. In reaction to the forces applied to it, bone grows. Your bones therefore become stronger as a result of lifting more weight. Additionally, it improves force output to sustain the strength of your spine, hips, and shoulders, allowing your entire body to function better well into old age.

TRY this simple dumbbell circuit: With a single dumbbell, perform ten squats, ten dumbbell rows on each arm, and ten push-ups of your choosing. Finish the reps and immediately go on to the next exercise, performing three rounds. Between each round, take a one to two-minute break. Use two dumbbells or increase the weight of one to make it more difficult.

6. Kickboxing

Kickboxing is a fantastic method to reduce stress, build muscle, and burn calories! It's a full-body workout since your arms can execute powerful jabs, crosses, hooks, and uppercuts by using the force generated by your legs. Along with testing your endurance and coordination, it will also help you become a better athlete both inside and outside of the ring.

Kickboxing pumps up your heart and lungs while working your legs, core, and especially your obliques to new heights. However, it also aids in improving proprioception, balance, and coordination. It is, in fact, a mind-body workout of the highest caliber.

TRY these five kicking combinations from the DailyBurn: Do eight repetitions of each combination for as long as you can for a half-hour. As needed, take a nap. Play your go-to battle music and maintain your fortitude!

7. Whirling

Whether on a stationary bike or an actual bike, spinning is one of the finest methods to increase endurance and burn calories. Spinning is an excellent, low-impact weight-loss exercise that works the largest, strongest muscles in the body. Like strength training, using your largest muscles helps burn fat across your entire body by triggering the production of new muscles through hormones.

8. High-intensity interval training, or HIIT

HIIT exercises are by far some of the best methods for increasing your metabolism and burning calories. The nice thing is that there is no set length for these workouts. Even though some HIIT workouts are only 10 minutes long, they are only successful if you give them your all and push your body to the maximum. HIIT is effective in burning belly fat.

All along, form is crucial. Ryan states that maintaining proper form is crucial to preventing injuries, even when doing high-intensity motions. "Focus closer on completing the reps and sets accurately and building load securely, and less consideration regarding the heap/pressure or weight force."

Try a HIIT workout for 20 minutes to boost your metabolism.

9. Pulling a row

The rowing machine at your gym is one of the greatest pieces of strength and cardio equipment, so if you haven't utilized it, you should. You'll train your arms, back, hamstrings, quadriceps, glutes, and core with this full-body exercise that will have you perspiring profusely. Unlike what most people believe, your legs—not your arms—are primarily responsible for your rowing power. Pulling the grip toward your chest requires you to drive your legs back and contract your quads and glutes.

Combining the best aspects of strength and cardio training, rowing targets the hips and shoulders while also being an excellent weight-loss technique. You are exerting both your heart and lungs simultaneously. People often work at desk jobs, which causes our backs to become rounded. By expanding your shoulders, hips, and spine, rowing assists in reversing this.

TRY a 15-minute rowing routine: Warm up for 5 minutes, then row at a steady, slow pace. After that, increase your speed to a moderate 22 strokes per minute for five minutes. Cool down for five minutes to wrap up the workout.

10. Burpees

Burpees are a terrific movement to add to your schedule if you can leap and execute high-intensity activities. According to White, "burpees are a great way to burn calories, shed fat, and help in building muscle." "High-intensity exercises like burpees can burn up to 50% more fat than traditional strength training," according to the author. Burpees are also an effective full-body workout that doesn't require any special equipment and can help improve cardiovascular health in addition to aiding in weight loss.

Starting from an upright position, raise your hands above your head to complete a burpee. Then, leap up while keeping your hands above your head. After that, lower yourself to the ground and assume a plank position (push yourself farther by adding a push-up).

11. Elliptical

Be not misled by the elliptical machine! It may appear to be a simple device that you may use to spin your legs while reading a magazine or watching TV. However, you'll run out of breath if you work too hard and increase the resistance. It won't do much to ride the elliptical at a leisurely pace; the real magic arrives when the blood begins to pump and the lungs begin to function. To extend your abs and contract your upper body muscles, make sure you stand up straight. You can burn more calories by swinging your arms and using the handles.

Elliptical machines, which offer a lesser impact while preserving fitness, are an excellent way to continue losing weight while shielding your body from additional stress. "It's especially beneficial for returning to running after recovering from an injury or for helping prevent injury at the onset."

12. The StairMaster

A flight of stairs demands effort to ascend. This is because steps are meant to be brief, requiring you to use other muscles to raise your complete body, such as your calves, quadriceps, and glutes.

A fantastic method for strengthening the hamstrings, quadriceps, and glutes is the StairMaster. Your body stays strong and toned and your metabolism stays elevated when you work the largest and strongest muscles in your body. So the next time you're in the gym, consider using a StairMaster machine or climbing a flight of steps.

Aim for an all-out effort by starting at a comfortable, moderate pace and working your way up to a HIIT StairMaster workout.

13. Combat cords

A great, fuss-free method for getting a full-body strength and cardio workout is using battle ropes. Battle ropes, when used at a high intensity, will quickly raise your heart rate.
There's something very rewarding and enjoyable about continuously slamming hefty ropes. It eases any strain you've had over the course of the day and provides you with a feeling of progress as well as consuming the muscles and lungs in the best manner conceivable.

To use them correctly, stand with your feet shoulder-distance apart and grasp one end of the rope with each hand. As you alternately whip your arms to send waves down to the rope anchor, bow your knees slightly and keep your chest raised. Try varying the speed and direction of the movement by using one arm to whip more quickly and the other to forcefully slam the rope.

Attempt this 15-minute exercise: begin by moving your arms in opposite directions. Strive to keep these waves going for the next five minutes. Regarding intensity or speed, don't worry. Just make an effort to persevere. For two more rounds, try this. Take a minute off between each round.

14. Swimming

If the pounding sensation of jogging is too much for you, swimming is a great low-impact exercise that combines strength and cardio conditioning. Water creates resistance, which makes you use more muscles to move more quickly and consume oxygen more sensibly. Do you need more inspiration to go swimming? Since the natural temperature of your body is 98.6 degrees, just working out in water which is roughly 78 degrees helps you burn even more calories than you would on land. It battles to stay warm in the water by burning fat and calories.

Swimming works your entire body, including your arms, legs, and core, to help you stay afloat. This helps you gain strength and endurance.

15. Yoga

A great low-impact workout for losing weight is yoga. Research indicates that yoga can help reduce stress, and that elevated cortisol levels can contribute to weight gain. Furthermore, yoga improves coordination, strength, and flexibility. When combined with a healthy diet, a regular exercise routine can aid in your weight loss efforts. Join a power yoga class in a heated studio if you're seeking for an additional way to burn calories while practicing yoga. Power poses and quicker vinyasas will help you tone your body in addition to burning more calories as you sweat.

16. Pilates

Similar to yoga, pilates emphasizes strength rather than flexibility. According to White, it's a fantastic kind of exercise since difficult movements have many advantages, such as increased flexibility, balanced muscle strength, better control over your back and limbs, and mental health benefits. Additionally, it encourages "a stronger and more toned core, lower back, hips, and buttocks."

17. Interval instruction

Interval training, which involves alternating between brief bursts of high effort and intervals of lower intensity or rest, may be helpful if you're doing a lot of cardio (such as walking or jogging) but aren't seeing the desired effects. Why? Even while you're not exercising, your muscles continue to burn calories because of their metabolic activity.

One approach to maximize your calorie burn in a short amount of time and gain the benefits of strength and cardio training is to work out in intervals. It takes hours for your body to cool down after an exercise since the intensity causes your metabolism to reset at a higher pace. This is alluded to as abundance post-practice oxygen utilization or EPOC. This means that, in contrast to working out continuously at a moderate speed, you continue to burn calories long after your session is over.

Beyond the EPOC effect, intervals are a fantastic technique to support weight loss. A significant portion of weight reduction also stems from mental health issues. When using intervals, it's beneficial to focus on individual gains rather than just the whole workout after each repetition or round of exercise.

TRY IT: If you're exercising in 30-second bursts, perform the activity of your choice for 30 seconds every minute, followed by a 30-second break. You can extend this to 45 seconds of action followed by 15 seconds of rest as you go. Recall that you should be exerting yourself to the fullest at that period so that you are exhausted.

CHAPTER 8: MANAGING STRESS AND EMOTIONAL CONSUMPTION

Determining The Reasons Behind Emotional Eating

Finding better coping methods for emotional eating is a process that begins with knowing its causes, which is something that many of us can relate to. Here's a summary of some typical causes for why individuals reach for food during emotional times:

Stress Overload: It's normal to turn to food for solace when life becomes too much. When faced with stressful situations, such as a demanding workday, familial strife, or everyday anxiety, reaching for food might offer some solace.

Emotional Turmoil: Handling intense feelings such as rage, loneliness, or despair can be very difficult. When we're depressed, food can become a means for us to escape those emotions or fill a hole.

Social Situations: Get-togethers and social occasions can be emotional eating minefields. The temptation to overeat can be great for a variety of reasons, such as feeling self-conscious in front of others, giving in to peer pressure, or utilizing food as a coping mechanism for social anxiety.

Past Trauma: Emotional eating can occasionally be the result of deeper problems arising from traumatic or trying experiences in the past. Eating can develop into a coping strategy for handling unresolved grief or traumatic experiences.

Body Image Issues: A lot of us struggle with our complicated relationships with our bodies, and emotional eating can be greatly influenced by bad body image. Feelings of uneasiness or discontent can momentarily subside when one turns to food for solace or stress alleviation.

Habit and Routine: Even though we're not consciously aware of the emotions causing the behavior, emotional eating might eventually become a habit or a routine reaction to particular triggers or circumstances.

Biochemical Factors: Because our bodies and brains are intricate, biological elements such as neurotransmitter imbalances or hormone swings can affect how we feel about food and how we eat.

Environmental Influences: Emotional eating may also be influenced by the surroundings in which we live. Our environment can influence the foods we eat, whether it's through regular exposure to food commercials, easy access to high-calorie snacks, or cultural norms surrounding eating and food.

Lack of Coping Skills: For some people, emotional eating is just the outcome of not knowing how to effectively manage stress, emotions, or challenging circumstances. It can seem simplest to turn to food when we have no other means of expressing our emotions.

diets and Restriction: Ironically, efforts to manage our food through restrictive diets frequently backfire and result in emotional eating episodes. Emotional eating can occur when a person feels cheated or guilty about their dietary choices, which can lead them to struggle against their limitations.

Cultural Influences: Our connection with eating might be influenced by cultural customs and attitudes around food. Emotional eating behaviors may arise, for instance, from the usage of food in some cultures as a symbol of celebration or love.

Lack of Awareness: Emotional eating can occasionally become so embedded in our routines that we aren't even aware that we are engaging in it. Eating carelessly when preoccupied or turning to food as a coping mechanism for discomfort or boredom are frequent occurrences.

Instant Gratification: Eating can bring comfort and pleasure right away, which makes it a tempting temporary coping strategy. But this fleeting solace frequently gives way to regret or guilt later on, which feeds the vicious cycle of emotional eating.

Self-Sabotage: Some people may eat emotionally out of self-punishment or self-sabotage on a subconscious level. This may result from low self-esteem or the conviction that they don't deserve to be content or well.

Social Conditioning: Many of us learn early on to equate food with comfort or pleasure. For instance, offering comfort food when sad or rewarding good conduct with sweets might establish enduring connections between food and emotional fulfillment.

Lack of Coping Skills: Food can quickly become our go-to coping method if we haven't learned healthy ways to deal with stress, emotions, or boredom. Breaking free from emotional eating behaviors requires learning other coping mechanisms like exercise, meditation, or creative outlets.

Cycle of Shame: Emotional eating frequently results in feelings of guilt, shame, or failure. These negative emotions can then be handled by continuing emotional eating episodes. Self-acceptance and compassion are necessary to end this cycle.

Unmet Needs: Emotional eating may occasionally be a sign of unfulfilled psychological or emotional needs. For instance, we might turn to food to soothe ourselves and fill the vacuum when we're feeling alone or disconnected.

We may start addressing the underlying problems and figuring out healthy coping mechanisms for our emotions by being aware of these typical triggers for emotional eating. There are several techniques we can employ to escape the pattern of emotional eating, such as asking friends or experts for assistance, engaging in mindfulness and self-awareness exercises, or looking for other ways to relieve stress.

Using Techniques For Relaxation To Reduce Stress

Reducing stress levels with relaxation techniques is crucial for our general health. Here are a few quick and easy methods to decompress and wind down:

Breathe deeply: When you're feeling anxious, stop and pay attention to your breathing. Shut your eyes, take a deep breath via your nose, then release it gradually through your mouth. Feel the tension release after doing this a few times.

Stretch It Out: Mild stretching might aid in promoting relaxation and relieving muscle tension. Take a few minutes to stretch your neck, back, arms, and legs. It is quite relaxing and has an incredible sensation.

Take a Walk: Taking a stroll outside can significantly reduce your stress levels. Walking at the neighborhood park or around the block can provide you with some much-needed fresh air and physical activity, which can help elevate your mood and calm your thoughts.

Play some of your favorite relaxing songs and allow the sound to envelop you. Choose a relaxing and soul-soothing sound, be it jazz, classical, or ambient noises from nature.

Practice mindfulness: Being mindful involves paying attention to your thoughts and feelings without passing judgment on them and being present in the moment. Sit quietly for a few minutes and concentrate on your breathing or your body's feelings. It's an easy yet effective method of lowering tension and elevating relaxation.

Enjoy a Cup of Tea: Drinking a warm cup of tea has a very reassuring effect. Select a calming herbal infusion such as peppermint or chamomile, and enjoy each sip slowly.

Write in Your Journal: Keeping a journal can help you get insight into your stressors and release pent-up emotions. Take out a pen and notebook, and write whatever comes to mind on the page without any bias.

Take a Warm Bath: The ultimate indulgence in relaxation is a warm bath. To further aid in alleviating stress, mix in some Epsom salts or aromatic oils, then soak your worries away.

Take Up a Hobby: You can feel so much better when you are doing something you enjoy. Schedule time for enjoyable and relaxing activities, such as knitting, gardening, painting, or playing an instrument.

Connect with Loved Ones: Getting together with friends and family might help you feel happier and less stressed. Reaching out to loved ones for connection and support—whether via phone, video chat, or in-person visit—can make you feel more at ease and supported.

Practice Gratitude: Give some thought to the things you have to be thankful for. This little exercise can improve your mood and make you feel calmer and happier.

Visualization: Shut your eyes and picture yourself in a calm, beautiful setting. Imagine everything, including the sights, sounds, and scents, and permit yourself to lose yourself completely in this peaceful mental picture.

Laugh Aloud: The best treatment is, in fact, laughter! Take in a humorous film, give a comedy podcast a try, or just hang out with someone who always makes you laugh. Laughter is a natural way to release endorphins, which reduce stress.

Engage Your Senses: To help you stay in the present, use your senses. Observe your surroundings' sights, sounds, tastes, smells, and textures. You can feel more grounded and less stressed and anxious by doing this.

Disconnect from Technology: Take a little break from screens and turn off all electronics for the day. After turning off your computer, phone, and TV, take some time to reflect quietly or partake in offline activities.

Progressive relaxation involves tensing and then releasing each muscle group in your body starting at your toes and working your way up. This method can aid in deep relaxation and the removal of bodily stress.

Appreciate Nature: Get outside and establish a connection with the natural world. Nature has a way of relieving stress and uplift, whether you're hiking, lounging in a park, or just taking in a flower's beauty.

Aromatherapy: Several smells, including jasmine, chamomile, and lavender, are thought to have relaxing effects. To bring these calming scents into your home, use sachets, candles, or essential oils.

Exercise Self-Compassion: Take care of oneself with kindness and self-compassion. Show yourself the same consideration and compassion that you would show a friend in need. This can support emotional health and lessen stress-related symptoms.

Seek Professional Assistance: Don't be afraid to get help from a mental health professional if stress and worry are having a major negative influence on your day-to-day activities. You can enhance your general well-being and manage stress more effectively by using the skills and strategies that therapy, counseling, or other professional support services can offer you.

Keep in mind that everyone has a different definition of relaxation, so figure out what suits you the most and include it in your daily routine. Managing stress and preserving your general health and well-being depend on you taking care of yourself.

Developing Healthy Coping Mechanisms Without Food

Finding healthy coping mechanisms for stress and emotions other than turning to food is essential for our general well-being. The following are some useful tactics you can attempt:

Keep Moving: Physical activity is a great approach to reduce stress and improve your mood. Find activities that you enjoy doing and incorporate them into your routine, whether it's going for a walk outside, a dance class, or a run.

Practice mindfulness: When faced with stress, mindfulness practices such as meditation or deep breathing can help you remain composed and in the moment. Every day, set aside a short period to sit still, concentrate on your breathing, and let go of all concerns and distractions.

Talk It Out: If you're feeling overwhelmed, get in touch with a friend, relative, or therapist. Just talking about your problems can sometimes relieve stress and offer insightful insight and support.

Locate Creative Outlets: Take part in creative expression activities, such as writing, drawing, cooking, or performing music. Using creativity as a healthy outlet can help you process your emotions and manage your stress.

Take Care of Yourself: Give yourself the attention it deserves by getting enough rest, eating healthily, and setting aside time for rest and rejuvenation. Meeting your emotional and physical requirements can help you maintain your resilience and be able to handle stress more effectively.

Establish Boundaries: Develop the ability to say no to requests that sap your vitality or cause needless stress in your life. An essential component of self-care is establishing boundaries with other people and putting your health first.

Practice Gratitude: Every day, set aside some time to consider your blessings. Reducing stress and changing your viewpoint can be achieved by concentrating on the positive aspects of your life.

Develop a toolkit of coping mechanisms that you find effective, such as gradual muscle relaxation, deep breathing, or visualization. Possessing an array of tactics at your disposal can aid in improving your stress management skills.

Keep in Touch: Keep in touch with your loved ones and friends, even if it's simply over the phone or via video chat. Having social support is crucial for stress management and preserving emotional health.

Take Part in Your Hobbies: Invest time in pursuits that you find enjoyable and fulfilling. Hobbies, whether they be crafting, gardening, or performing an instrument, can help you feel fulfilled and divert your attention from stress.

Practice Relaxation Techniques: Try out several methods of relaxation, such as utilizing essential oils for aromatherapy, taking a warm bath, or listening to relaxing music. Make it a habit to incorporate your go-to method for relaxation into your self-care regimen.

Concentrate on the Present: Use grounding or mindfulness exercises to practice remaining in the present moment. Let go of concerns about the past or the future, pay attention to your environment, and pay attention to the feelings in your body.

Express Yourself: Whether it's by writing in a notebook, speaking with a reliable friend, or using artistic expression, discover healthy ways to communicate your feelings. You can process emotions and lower your stress level by expressing your sentiments.

Reduce Stressful Triggers: Recognize the sources of stress in your life and, if at all possible, reduce or eliminate them. This could entail assigning duties to others, prioritizing chores, or defining boundaries with particular persons or circumstances.

Practice Self-Compassion: Be nice and compassionate to yourself, especially when things are tough. Remember to treat yourself with kindness and acknowledge that it's normal to experience moments of tension or exhaustion.

Emphasis on Healthy Coping Mechanisms: Rather than consuming comfort food, concentrate on assembling a toolkit of constructive coping techniques. This could involve reading, listening to music, going outside, or engaging in mindfulness exercises.

obtain Plenty of Rest: To maintain your physical and mental well-being, make it a priority to obtain enough sleep every night. Sleep deprivation can increase stress and make it more difficult to handle difficult situations.

Exercise Persistence and Patience: Recall that effective stress management is a journey, and it's acceptable to make incremental changes in your behavior. Be kind to yourself and acknowledge your accomplishments as you go.

Seek Professional Assistance: Don't be afraid to ask for support from a therapist or counselor if you're finding it difficult to manage your stress on your own. They can provide you with more resources and techniques to help you deal with challenging feelings and circumstances.

It's acceptable to seek assistance when necessary, and developing constructive coping mechanisms for stress requires patience and experience. As you experiment with several tactics and determine which one suits you the best, practice self-compassion.

CHAPTER 9: PRIORITIZING SLEEP FOR EFFECTIVE WEIGHT LOSS

Understanding The Connection Between Sleep And Losing Weight.

Have you ever noticed that your appetite seems to go into overdrive when you don't get enough sleep? It turns out that this is due to a scientific explanation. Our bodies create more of the hormone ghrelin, which alerts our brain to hunger, and less of the hormone leptin, which alerts our brains to fullness when we are sleep-deprived. It may be more difficult to maintain a healthy diet and lose weight as a result of this imbalance since it can boost cravings and overindulge.

However, it goes beyond simply being hungry. We are also less likely to have the drive or energy to exercise when we are sleepy. Not only does sleep deprivation interfere with our metabolism, but it also seems as though our body is telling us, "Why go for a run when you could just take a nap?"

The worst part is that our bodies are more inclined to retain fat when we don't get enough sleep, especially around our bellies. This is because insufficient sleep can create hormone disruption and insulin resistance, which facilitates the body's tendency to store fat rather than metabolize it for energy.

Not only do our hunger hormones get imbalanced when we don't get enough sleep. Additionally, when our bodies experience increased stress, the stress hormone cortisol may rise as a result. In addition to making us feel more tense and nervous, elevated cortisol levels can also cause cravings for foods heavy in fat and sugar. Thus, it's like getting two benefits for trying to lose weight.

Furthermore, a lack of sleep impairs our bodies' ability to metabolize glucose, which can result in insulin resistance and, eventually, weight gain. In addition, sleep deprivation can impair our ability to control our impulses and make it more difficult to resist a late-night snack or a second helping of dessert.

Therefore, getting enough sleep is just as crucial for weight loss as eating a healthy diet and exercising. Here are a few easy suggestions to improve your quality of sleep:

Even on weekends, maintain a regular sleep routine by going to bed and waking up at the same time each day.

Establish a calming nighttime routine to let your body know when it's time to unwind. This can entail activities like reading a book, doing deep breathing exercises or having a warm bath.

Make sure your bedroom is quiet, dark, and cold so that you can sleep well.

Reduce the amount of time you spend on screens before bed since the blue light from computers, tablets, and phones can disrupt your body's normal circadian rhythm.

Stay away from caffeine and large meals right before bed because they can cause sleep disturbances.

Engage in regular exercise during the day, but try to avoid doing strenuous activity right before bed.

Use stress-reduction methods like yoga, meditation, or journaling to help you relax and get a better night's sleep.

Establish a Comfortable Sleep Environment: Ensure that your bedroom is a conducive place to sleep. To reduce distractions, choose a cozy mattress and cushions and think about using a white noise machine or blackout curtains.

Limit Your Alcohol Consumption: Although a nightcap may make you fall asleep more quickly, it can also interfere with your sleep cycles and reduce the quality of your sleep in general. Limit your alcohol intake in the hours before going to bed.

Practice Relaxation Techniques: To help you relax and get your body ready for sleep, include relaxation techniques like progressive muscle relaxation, guided imagery, or meditation in your nightly routine.

Limit Naps: Taking naps throughout the day can disrupt your sleep cycle at night, even if a quick snooze can be revitalizing. Aim to avoid naps too close to bedtime and limit naps to 20 to 30 minutes.

Maintain a Balanced Diet: Eating a healthy diet might help you sleep better as well. Caffeine, sugary snacks, and large or spicy meals should be avoided in the hours before bed as these can interfere with sleep.

Get Some Sunlight During the Day: Being exposed to daylight during the day helps your body's internal clock to be more in sync with the nighttime sleep cycle. Make an effort to get outside every day, preferably in the early.

Seek expert Assistance if Needed: Don't be afraid to ask for advice from a healthcare expert if you've done everything and are still having trouble falling asleep. They can offer tailored advice for enhancing the quality of your sleep as well as assist in identifying any underlying sleep disorders or problems.

You may enhance your general health and well-being as well as help your weight reduction objectives by giving sleep a higher priority and implementing a few easy changes to your bedtime routine.

Making A Nighttime Routine To Improve The Quality Of Your Sleep

Now, let's discuss creating a daily schedule that will improve your quality of sleep. Consider it your wind-down period, when you're setting your body and mind up for a restful night.

Regular Bedtime: Make an effort to go to bed and wake up at roughly the same time each day. Although it may seem uninteresting, following a schedule aids in regulating your internal clock because your body thrives on routine.

Unwind Before Bed: Allow yourself to unwind for at least thirty to sixty minutes before going to bed. Instead of using screens, choose peaceful pursuits like reading a book, having a warm bath, or performing some gentle stretching.

Check Your Screen Time: Speaking of screens, try not to use them an hour before going to bed. That means no Netflix binge-watching in bed or thumbing through your phone. Screen blue light disrupts sleep hormones, making it more difficult to fall asleep.

Comfortable Bedroom Ambience: Create a haven of rest in your bedroom. Make sure the space is calm, dark, and cold, and get comfortable bedding that will lull you to sleep.

Reduce Your Stimulants: Avoid caffeine and nicotine in the evening as they act as tiny sleep disruptors. Although a nightcap may seem soothing, it's advised to avoid alcohol as it can interfere with your sleep cycles.

Create a nightly routine that signals to your body that it is time to relax. Whatever works for you—drinking herbal tea, stretching lightly, or writing down your thoughts in a journal—find a bedtime routine and stick with it.

Maintain Your Good Sleep Habits: Don't let them slip. A comfortable mattress and pillows, a tidy and clutter-free bedroom, and a regular sleep regimen all contribute to higher-quality sleep.

Light Dinner: Steer clear of large, spicy meals right before bed. It can be difficult to fall asleep after eating a large dinner too late because it will make you feel bloated and uncomfortable.

Stress management: Before going to bed, find techniques to relax and reduce tension. A brief moment of relaxation, whether it be through deep breathing exercises, relaxing music, or a brief meditation, can significantly improve the quality of your sleep.

Limit Daytime Naps: Despite the allure of a fast power nap, avoid sleeping for extended periods during the day. It may interfere with your sleep cycle and make it more difficult for you to fall asleep at night.

Establish a Cozy and Inviting Sleep Environment: Make sure your bedroom is a comfortable place to stay. To help you sleep, get comfortable, breathable bedding, and think about adding white noise machines or blackout curtains to block out any disturbances.

Unwind with Calm Activities: Engage in peaceful, stress-relieving activities before going to bed. This might be anything from meditating or doing mild yoga to sipping a warm cup of herbal tea devoid of caffeine.

Reduce Liquid Intake Before Bed: Try to reduce the amount of liquids you consume in the hours before bed to help you prevent having to wake up in the middle of the night to use the restroom. This can assist you in getting uninterrupted, better sleep.

Modify Lighting: To tell your body it's time to relax, dim the lights in your house in the evening. To create a comfortable and relaxing ambiance, think about employing soft, warm-toned lighting.

Establish a Bedtime Routine: Make sure you have a nightly schedule that you stick to. This can entail doing things like cleaning your face, brushing your teeth, and reading a book in bed. To tell your body when it's time to go to sleep, you must be consistent.

Practice Gratitude: Before going to bed, take time to consider your blessings. Before going to bed, practicing thankfulness might help you turn your attention from pressures and problems and encourage a more upbeat outlook.

Reduce Your Exposure to Upsetting Content: Before going to bed, steer clear of anything emotionally charged or upsetting to read or watch. Instead, choose upbeat and peaceful media that promotes relaxation and helps you decompress.

Try your hand at aromatherapy: To create a calming atmosphere in your bedroom, try using essential oils like chamomile or lavender. To encourage relaxation and better sleep, you can apply these oils physically, diffuse them, or mix them into a warm bath.

Make a Calm Bedtime Playlist: Before going to bed, make a playlist of soothing songs or sounds of the natural world. Playing soothing music might help you relax and get ready for a good night's sleep.

Remain Calm and Patient: It takes time and patience to build good sleeping habits. Maintain consistency in your nighttime routine and don't give up if you don't see benefits right away. Continue trying out various tactics until you determine which one suits you the best.

You'll be well on your way to better sleep and all the advantages that go along with it, like enhanced mood, sharper focus, and a happier, healthier you, if you include these suggestions into your nighttime routine.

Changing Your Sleeping Surroundings To Improve Your Quality Of Sleep

Let's discuss how to create a comfortable haven in your bedroom for restful sleep.

Get Comfortable: How well you sleep is greatly influenced by your mattress and pillows. It could be time for an upgrade if your pillows are worn out or your mattress is bumpy and ancient. To make it easier for you to fall asleep, choose supportive and cozy bedding.

Shut Off the Light: Have you ever noticed how even a tiny amount of light coming in through the curtains can cause sleep disturbances? Invest in blackout blinds or curtains to maintain a dark and cozy space. If that isn't an option, consider blocking off distracting light with a sleep mask.

Keep it cold: It's critical to have a cold bedroom because sleeping causes your body temperature to naturally drop. The ideal sleeping temperature is between 60 and

67°F (15 and 19°C). Try different bedding fabrics to see what will keep you warm without being too hot.

Please be quiet. If you reside in a noisy neighborhood, noise can seriously interfere with your ability to sleep. To block out undesirable noise, think about utilizing white noise generators or earplugs. Some people find that relaxing noises, such as the sound of the ocean or rain, can make it easier for them to fall asleep.

Get Rid of the Clutter: It can be difficult to unwind and get asleep when there is clutter in the bedroom or the head. Spend some time organizing your room and setting up a relaxing atmosphere. It will not only improve your quality of sleep, but it will also make mornings a little more enjoyable.

Establish a peaceful Atmosphere: Dim lighting, mellow hues, and comforting aromas can all aid in establishing a peaceful environment that promotes sleep. To transform your bedroom into a haven, think about adding accessories like throw blankets, candles, and essential oils.

Unplug before going to bed: The blue light that electronics emit might interfere with your body's normal circadian rhythm, making it more difficult to fall asleep. Before going to bed, try to avoid using screens for at least an hour. Instead, choose relaxing activities like reading a book or taking a bath.

Create a Routine: By establishing a nightly schedule, you can tell your body when it's time to relax and get ready for slumber. Find a bedtime routine that works for you, whether it's brushing your teeth, stretching, or simply drinking a cup of herbal tea.

Invest in High-Quality Bedding: Give yourself a luxurious set of warm blankets and silky sheets that will make you eager to get into bed every night. The quality of your bedding can have a significant impact on your level of comfort and sleep quality.

Think About Your Mattress: A comfortable mattress is the cornerstone of a restful night's sleep, so pick one based on your preferences and needs. Take your time to choose the ideal mattress for you, whether you like a firm or softer feel.

Add Some Greenery: Adding a little bit of nature to your bedroom might help make it feel more peaceful. Think about bringing in a few air-purifying houseplants to liven up your interior while also adding some greenery.

Choose Your Bedroom Color Wisely: Colors can significantly affect your mood and the quality of your sleep. For a calm atmosphere that promotes relaxation, go for calming, neutral colors like earthy neutrals, gentle blues, or greens.

Establish a Tech-Free Zone: When you're winding down for the night, keep electronics out of the bedroom or at least out of reach. Screen blue light might interfere with your sleep cycle and make it more difficult to fall asleep.

Create a Wind-Down Routine: Schedule some time each night to de-stress and unwind before going to bed. Discover hobbies that assist you in calming down from the stress of the day, such as light yoga, reading a book, or having a warm bath.

Employ aromatherapy: Fragrances such as vanilla, chamomile, and lavender are well known for their calming effects and can aid in improving sleep quality. To bring these calming scents into your bedroom, try using essential oils or a diffuser.

Maintain Silence: To filter out unpleasant noises in your bedroom, think about using earplugs or a white noise machine. To absorb sound and create a calmer space, you can also consider laying heavy curtains or rugs.

Optimize Your Sleep Position: Try a variety of postures to see which one suits you the best. Regardless of your preferred sleeping position—on your side, back, or stomach—be sure your mattress and pillow are supporting your neck and spine enough.

Take Care of Allergens: Dust mites and pet dander are two allergens that can seriously impair your quality of sleep. If you are allergic to anything, make sure your bedroom is dust-free and clean, and think about using hypoallergenic bedding.

Eliminate Clock-Watching: Continually glancing at the time can exacerbate anxiety and interfere with sleep. To help you relax and fall asleep more quickly, think about moving clocks out of your bedroom or turning them so they are not in your direct line of sight.

Above all, pay attention to what makes you sleep better and pay attention to your body. Since every person has distinct sleep demands, try out a variety of methods and approaches until you determine which ones are most effective for you.

You may improve your chances of getting a better night's sleep and waking up feeling rejuvenated and prepared to take on the day by designing a sleep-friendly environment that suits your requirements and preferences.

CHAPTER 10: GETTING PAST CHALLENGES

Handling The Irksome Periods When Your Weight Loss Stops

Although it can be quite discouraging, many of us encounter weight loss plateaus when trying to adopt healthier lifestyles. Here are some helpful hints to get you through those frustrating periods when you feel like your weight loss is stagnating:

Breathe, Look Back: It's important to stand back and consider your progress when you reach a plateau. Think back on your progress and the constructive adjustments you've made to your way of life. It's important to consider not only the weight on the scale but also the advancements you've made in your overall health and well-being.

Change Up Your Routine: Your body may have grown accustomed to your food and workout regimen if you have been following them for a long. Change things up by doing new exercises, combining various forms of physical activity, or experimenting in the kitchen with new, healthful foods. In addition to helping people overcome plateaus, variety keeps things engaging and pleasurable.

Pay Attention to Non-Scale Victories: Occasionally, your accomplishments go unnoticed by the scale. Celebrate other successes, like as gains in strength, endurance, vitality, and general well-being, rather than concentrating just on the number on the scale. These intangible successes are equally significant and can sustain your motivation when you hit a plateau.

Remain Consistent: Overcoming plateaus in the weight loss process requires consistency, yet plateaus are a normal part of the journey. Maintain your healthy lifestyle even if you're not experiencing effects right away. Even if your positive decisions don't immediately reflect on the scale, keep in mind that every choice you make is a step in the right direction.

Be Aware of Portions: Oftentimes, we don't even realize when our portion sizes are increasing. Keep an eye on portion sizes and practice mindfulness when eating. To help you reduce portion sizes, keep track of how much food you eat and think about using smaller dishes and plates.

Keep Yourself Hydrated: Drinking lots of water promotes general health and aids in weight loss. Our body might sometimes misinterpret thirst for hunger, causing us to eat when we're simply dehydrated. To stay hydrated during the day, try to drink eight glasses of water or more each day and carry a water bottle around with you.

Handle Stress: Stress can cause physical harm to our bodies and impede weight loss efforts. Discover healthy coping mechanisms for stress, such as mindfulness training, deep breathing techniques, or enjoying enjoyable hobbies. It's critical to look after your emotional and physical health on par with your physical health.

Get Enough Sleep: Sleep deprivation can interfere with hormone balance and metabolism, making weight loss more difficult. Aim for seven to nine hours of healthy sleep every night and give proper sleep hygiene habits, such as planning a regular sleep schedule and a calming nighttime routine, priority.

Above all, remember to be patient and optimistic toward yourself. Always keep in mind that losing weight is a journey with ups and downs. Honor all of your accomplishments, no matter how tiny, and try not to be too hard on yourself when you reach a plateau. Have faith in the procedure and proceed cautiously, one step at a time.

Track Your Progress: You can keep track of your food intake, exercise routine, and general progress by keeping a journal or utilizing a tracking app. Seeing the results of your labors in front of you can inspire you and provide you insight into potential areas for improvement.

Boost Physical Activity: Increasing your level of physical activity may help you break through a weight loss stall. This may be finding methods to be more active throughout the day, such as walking or using the stairs instead of the elevator, adding an extra workout session, or increasing the intensity of your workouts every week.

Review Your Objectives: Give your objectives a second look to see if they're still reasonable and attainable. To stay motivated and focused on your success, think about setting new goals if some of your early ones have already been attained.

Seek Support: If you're feeling stuck, don't be scared to ask friends, family, or a medical expert for assistance. Establishing a support network can help you stay on track toward your objectives by offering accountability, encouragement, and insightful counsel.

Think About Professional Advice: If, despite your best efforts, you've been unable to overcome a plateau, you might want to consult a personal trainer, certified dietitian, or other healthcare professional for advice. They can provide you with individualized guidance and encouragement to get beyond setbacks and accomplish your weight loss objectives.

You may overcome weight loss plateaus and keep moving in the direction of a healthier, happier you by putting these techniques into practice and maintaining your focus on your objectives. Remain confident in yourself and never forget that you can accomplish incredible things!

Trying New Strategies To Quicken Your Progress

Trying some new strategies can be the perfect way to get your weight reduction journey back on track if you're feeling stuck. Here are some doable suggestions to change things up and hasten your progress:

Change Up Your Meals: To keep your meals interesting and fulfilling, try out new recipes and ingredients. Changing up your diet and making healthy eating more pleasurable can be achieved by experimenting with different fruits, vegetables, grains, and proteins.

Move Your Body in Novel Ways: Experiment with diverse workouts to shake up your fitness regimen. Finding things you enjoy will help keep you active and less like a job. Some examples of these activities include dancing, hiking, swimming, and trying out different fitness classes.

Eating with awareness: Develop mindful eating by being aware of your body's signals of hunger and fullness. Take your time, enjoy every meal, and pay attention to the feelings that certain cuisines evoke in you. This can assist you in creating a more positive relationship with food and in making more deliberate decisions.

Remain Hydrated: To keep hydrated and assist your body's natural functions, make sure you drink lots of water throughout the day. You can enhance the taste and appeal of your water by adding fruit or herb pieces.

receive Quality Sleep: To help you in your weight loss attempts, make sure you receive adequate sleep every night. To help you decompress and get ready for sleep, establish a calming nighttime ritual and aim for seven to nine hours of excellent sleep.

Find Support: Make connections with loved ones, close friends, or a support group so that they can encourage and cheer you on as you go. Having a solid support network can help you remain accountable and motivated.

Honor Non-Scale Wins: Keep in mind that development isn't solely determined by a scale's number. Honor other accomplishments, such as having more energy, downsizing in size, or choosing better options all day long.

Remain Positive: Remain upbeat and concentrate on the accomplishments you've made, no matter how modest. There will inevitably be ups and downs on any weight reduction journey, but staying optimistic will keep you resilient and motivated when things become hard.

Listen to Your Body: Be aware of your body's reactions to various foods and activities, and modify your strategy accordingly. The best advice is to listen to your body's cues and make decisions that promote your general health and well-being.

Be Patient: Keep in mind that long-term, sustainable weight loss requires patience and that there will unavoidably be ups and downs. Remain constant in your efforts, have patience with yourself, and have faith that your efforts will eventually be rewarded.

You may overcome obstacles, maintain your motivation, and move closer to your objectives by implementing these techniques into your weight loss journey. Continue experimenting, be devoted, and don't forget to acknowledge and appreciate your small victories along the way!

Keeping Motivation And Optimism In The Face Of Difficulty

It can be quite difficult to maintain your motivation and optimism when things are difficult. However, the following practical advice might be useful:

Accept it One Step at a Time: Try dividing large activities into smaller, more doable ones when you feel overwhelmed. Instead of attempting to do everything at once, concentrate on taking one task at a time.

Find the Silver Linings: Usually, there is something good to be found, even in the worst of circumstances. Pause for a moment and consider what you have to be thankful for or what you might be learning from the experience.

Rely on Your Support Network: Don't be scared to ask for help from friends, family, or even online communities. Having a conversation with a caring person can often have a profound impact.

Permit Yourself to Feel: When things don't go your way, it's acceptable to experience frustration, sadness, or anger. Remember that feeling such things is a natural part of being human, and permit yourself to feel them without passing judgment.

Take Care of Yourself: Even in difficult times, remember to give self-care priority. Do whatever makes you feel renewed and invigorated—whether it's cuddling up with a good book, taking a bubble bath, or taking a stroll around the park.

Continue Pushing Forward: Try not to give up, even if it's only a little bit each day, and don't give up if things seem to be going slowly or you're having difficulties. Never forget that any action, no matter how tiny, is still a positive move.

Seek Out Positive: Be in the company of positive and inspiring people. Find positive things to do whenever you can, whether it's watching a hilarious movie, listening to your favorite music, or spending time with loved ones.

Celebrate Your Wins: Regardless of how minor they may appear, give yourself permission to recognize and honor your accomplishments. Give yourself a pat on the back for a job well done, whether it's finishing a task, hitting a goal, or just making it through a difficult day.

Remain Adaptable: Recognize that things don't always go as planned and accept that. If things don't go as planned, don't be too hard on yourself, and be prepared to modify your expectations and goals as necessary.

Last but not least, have faith in yourself. You are more resilient and strong than you may think. Have faith in your ability to manage any situation that arises, and know that you possess the fortitude and inner fortitude to conquer even the most difficult obstacles.

Above all, remember to treat yourself with kindness and allow yourself the grace to persevere, show compassion, and be resilient throughout trying times.

CHAPTER 11: GETTING HELP WHEN REQUIRED

Mentioning Support From Friends And Family, Companions, Or Web Gatherings.

Loved ones can assume an essential part in supporting and adding to an individual's weight reduction venture. The following are multiple ways they can help:

Consistent reassurance: Weight reduction can be testing both actually and inwardly. Loved ones can give support, inspiration, and understanding during troublesome times. They can offer a listening ear, celebrate victories, and give a positive climate.

Responsibility accomplices: Having somebody to consider you responsible can essentially affect your weight reduction endeavors. Loved ones can check in routinely, screen progress, and assist you with keeping focused with your objectives. This should be possible through standard gatherings, calls, or utilizing versatile applications that track progress.

Practice mates: Finding a companion or relative who shares your wellness objectives can make practice more charming and increment inspiration. You can work out together, join wellness classes or sports exercises, or essentially take strolls or runs. Having an exercise accomplice can make the cycle more tomfoolery and offer extra help.

Solid preparing and feast arranging: Loved ones can uphold your weight reduction venture by participating in sound preparing and dinner arranging exercises. They can help exploration and offer nutritious recipes, cook good feasts together, or even alternate facilitating solid supper gatherings. Furthermore, they can energize better food decisions while eating out or going to get-togethers.

Dynamic social exercises: Rather than zeroing in exclusively on food-focused social exercises, loved ones can recommend and partake in dynamic trips. This could incorporate climbing, trekking, moving, playing sports, or arranging bunch exercises like forager chases or wellness challenges. Integrating proactive tasks into parties advances a functioning way of life.

Eliminating enticements: Loved ones can help by establishing a strong climate. This includes eliminating or limiting the presence of unfortunate food sources in shared spaces, shunning offering enticing treats, and regarding dietary decisions. Having a strong climate at home and during parties can make it simpler to adhere to good dieting propensities.

Training and assets: Loved ones can help by giving instructive materials, and suggesting enlightening books, web recordings, or narratives about sound living and weight reduction. They can share their insight and encounters, keeping you educated and roused on your excursion.

Praising achievements: Celebrating weight reduction achievements and accomplishments is significant. Loved ones can recognize your advancement and express pride in your achievements. This encouraging feedback can support certainty and inspiration to forge ahead with the weight reduction venture.
Keep in mind, it's fundamental to impart your requirements and objectives with your friends and family to guarantee they comprehend how best to help you on your weight reduction venture. Everybody's process is interesting, and their help can be custom-made to your particular necessities.

Online gatherings
Another choice that doesn't need face to face gatherings includes online help discussions. Most discussions offer a protected spot for individuals to share stories as well as diet and exercise plans, in addition to look for inspiration.

Models include:
Bariatric Buddy
Heftiness Help
3 Fat Chicks on a Tight eating routine

Remember, however, that a significant number individuals on these gatherings aren't clinical experts and may offer you wrong counsel. Continuously check with a specialist prior to beginning another eating regimen plan or exercise program.

Applications

Weight reduction applications are unquestionably valuable. They can assist you with following your calorie admission and exercise. Large numbers of them likewise offer help as online entertainment associations and discussion channels.

For instance, the application MyFitnessPal has a message discussion where you can interface with different clients to share tips and examples of overcoming adversity.

The application for the wearable wellness sensor Fitbit likewise has solid local area highlights. When you buy a Fitbit watch, you can interface with different loved ones who likewise have a Fitbit. You can take part in difficulties with them and even find a nearby test with individuals you don't have the foggiest idea.

One more application known as FatSecret permits you to visit with others and make or join gatherings to interface with individuals who have comparable objectives.

Finding a Responsibility Accomplice

What is a responsibility accomplice?
A responsibility accomplice is somebody who understands what your objectives are and will consider you responsible to guarantee that you get to where you need to be. Basically, where you'd regularly pull off skirting a Monday morning run, a weight reduction accomplice would know regardless of whether you had done what you set off on a mission to do - so there's no stowing away!

While this could sound a piece overwhelming, it very well may be truly tomfoolery and persuading. A weight reduction responsibility accomplice might be working close by you to arrive at comparative objectives, so you can uphold each other on your excursion to getting more fit. Consider them your greatest team promoter who you can direct consequently.

What are the advantages of having a weight reduction responsibility accomplice?

At last, a weight reduction responsibility accomplice will have an instrumental impact in your emotionally supportive network and help you on your excursion to shedding weight. Imparting your experience to another mate, huge other, or relative will make it that additional piece simpler and energizing. Here are only a couple of justifications for why you ought to consider finding a weight reduction accomplice or joining a weight reduction pal framework:

They'll inspire you through consolation - Practicing alone may not generally be a tomfoolery ride, but rather you can anticipate meetups with your weight reduction accomplice.

They can offer you their recommendation - if at any point you're in uncertainty, this individual can offer you their help. Attempt to continuously tell the truth and speak with one another plainly so that you're both mindful of each other's circumstance.

You can share achievement - you'll both be on a weight reduction venture so it will be remunerating to see each other succeed and you'll have somebody to celebrate with.

They'll assist you with remaining focused - having somebody to check in with and screen your advancement implies you'll be more averse to lead astray.

You'll have the option to help them as well - this organization will work the two different ways, so you'll get a genuine deep satisfaction when you see your accomplice shedding pounds as well.

Step by step instructions to be a decent responsibility accomplice

Keep in mind, by finding a responsibility accomplice, you will end up being a responsibility accomplice yourself; a relationship works the two different ways. In light of this, we've assembled a few top ways to be a mindful responsibility accomplice to guarantee that you both arrive at your maximum capacity.

1. Put forth yourselves Brilliant objectives

Before you and your weight reduction amigo get to chip away at being more dynamic and eating great, ensure you set aside some margin to plunk down together and distinguish your key objectives. Your objectives ought to be Brilliant, which represents:

Explicit - "Practicing more" would be an extremely unclear objective. All things considered, consider how much activity you need to do every week or settle on precisely how much weight you both wish to lose.

Quantifiable - you ought to have the option to keep tabs on your development so ensure that you and your accomplice put forth quantifiable objectives. For example, assuming that you want to turn out for thirty minutes every day, you'll effectively have the option to screen this.

Reachable - be reasonable. Getting abs in seven days would be anybody's fantasy yet it isn't probably going to work out. All things being equal, put forth yourself more modest objectives and set new ones as you accomplish them.
Applicable - consider the justifications for why you and your accomplice wish to define the objectives you've picked. Having an explanation for the objective will end up being a genuine inspiration.

Time-bound - put it down on the calendar for you as well as your accomplice to arrive at your objectives as this will give you something to pursue.

2. Plan your exercises and feasts

By placing dates in the journal for exercises and arranging out your feasts for the week, you'll be bound to get practice in and adhere to your eating routine. Without an arrangement set up, you might find it trying to find times that suit both of you and pass up shared encounters.

3. Tell the truth

You must keep your weight reduction accomplice on target as well; be transparent with them so they also can arrive at their objectives. For instance, assuming they've missed the last two or three meetups to work out, delicately help them to remember their objective and urge them to stay on track. It very well might be an instance of returning to the arrangement you made together or re-defining a few objectives so that they're more practical. By imparting really, you can figure out the best methodology.

4. Make it fun

An extraordinary method for remaining inspired is to enliven your feasts and work-out schedules. In the event that you and your weight reduction responsibility accomplice wind up going on similar strolling trails or eating similar good feasts every week, you could without much of a stretch become exhausted.

You could likewise attempt to set a weight reduction pal challenge and make your meetings more serious. For instance, you could scrutinize your cardio by seeing who can do the most star hops in a single moment. Assuming your time together is more pleasant, you'll need to keep doing awesome!

5. Appear

Got another most loved Television program that you essentially can't miss or you're "simply not feeling it"? Remember that when you don't go up to a meeting, you're by all accounts not the only one who will be let down. Being liable for another person's prosperity as much as your own ought to fill you with inspiration, however you simply should be steady and try not to miss any meet-ups with your accomplice.

Definitely there will be events when you can't make an exercise meeting or end up enjoying food sources you committed to stay away from, yet you'll have to re-center and get back around track on the off chance that this occurs. Assuming that you're battling, your weight reduction accomplice will be there to help you.

6. Audit each other's advancement.

Remember to monitor one another and ensure that you're both still on target to arriving at your objectives. Maybe you'll choose to gauge yourselves toward the finish of every week and report back, logging your weight reduction. In the event that both of you observe that you're not losing however much weight that you'd trusted, you can hope to update your feast plans or how much activity you're doing every week.

7. Show restraint toward one another

You'll both be pushing each other out of your usual ranges of familiarity, so you'll likely hit a few snags or find the cycle testing on occasion. Make sure to continuously keep a positive, killer instinct and backing each other constantly.

8. Celebrate achievement!

At the point when you or your accomplice get in shape, ensure you celebrate (in a sound way!); regardless of whether you or your weight reduction mate lost only one pound, this is as yet a step in the right direction. While progress might appear delayed to begin with, the sets of you will before long start being more dynamic and eating better which will emphatically affect your general wellbeing.

Contemplating finding support from a mentor or guide

Diet and Exercise Alone Are adequately not

Purifies, detox programs, trend slims down, training camps, and numerous different endeavors have been started to assist with settling the issues of an overweight country. Certain individuals experience achievement while starting another eating routine system or an activity program. Be that as it may, a lot more don't. All things being equal, they experience sensations of disappointment and rout when they can't finish a program. A few people will find lasting success in finishing their projects and will get thinner, an impact the program is intended to assist them with accomplishing. Nonetheless, a significant number of these equivalent people will get back to past way of life propensities and endlessly, recover the weight and at times considerably more. In that lies the issue.

Change is Hard

Many individuals can adhere to another program or change for a set number of days realizing there will be the point at which the program is finished and they can continue their everyday living. These people will do whatever it takes, once in a while in outrageous ways, to meet a momentary objective. For instance, somebody on a 7-day purge will drink the suggested scrub beverages for those 7 days. In any case, when the period is finished, the individual continues their typical course of eating in light of the fact that the purify gives no suggestions or bearings for how to keep eating or drinking for a lifetime.

It's been said endlessly time once more, however maybe it merits expressing here something like again. The best change that happens for any individual needing to roll out enduring improvements, is a way of life change. This requires the individual to not just recognize parts in their day to day existence that need to change yet additionally to have the limit and capacity to rehearse these progressions day to day until the end of their life.

Little switches add around to large outcomes. Incidentally, the little changes and slow advancement individuals battle with the most. We are a country of speedy arrangements and moment delight, and when we don't see the outcomes or live up to our assumptions rapidly, our determination and confidence in the process fade. At last, we surrender and return to what is agreeable and what we know. This is where treatment can help.

What Kinds of Treatment Are Ideal?

Mental Social Treatment (CBT) is one of the most broadly utilized and embraced styles of treatment and is upheld in light of the fact that it is a proof based approach. "Proof based" signifies research has been led and information has been gathered to help and show this procedure takes care of business and results have demonstrated fruitful results.

CBT focuses on the methodology of recognizing dangerous idea designs (like negative contemplations) that might slow down or go against objectives. For instance, the idea, "Indeed, I've previously gobbled this treat and wrecked my eating routine at this point. Should simply eat a couple of more and refocus one week from now." This is an illustration of Go big or go home Reasoning. Using CBT systems, an instructor would assist the client with recognizing these contemplations and make centered intercessions to shut down these considerations, and in this way, stop the way of behaving (gorging on the treats).

Rationalistic Conduct Treatment (DBT) centers around distinguishing considerations and ways of behaving while at the same time looking for a method for understanding and acknowledge them without judgment. DBT is the possibility that an individual can have inverse contemplations and ways of behaving from various sides of the range, yet not have a need to transform them. Any other way, two inverse things can be valid simultaneously. For instance, an individual might battle with being overweight and need to get thinner, while simultaneously eating an eating routine that isn't helpful for weight reduction nevertheless be good with these realities. This individual would embrace and acknowledge they are a work underway and realize that change requires some investment.

This can engage the client battling with weight issues to turn out to be less critical of their entanglements with diet and objectives related with weight the board. DBT focuses on the utilization of care strategies, mindfulness, and taking part in certain adapting abilities like breathing procedures. DBT assists clients with finding self-acknowledgment and occupies from go big or go home, or high contrast thinking.

Wellbeing Training is one of the freshest and latest ways to deal with helping individuals in their weight the board plans. Wellbeing training is assisting people with ingraining solid propensities and systems into their day to day routines. Through training, people are upheld with everyday updates, inspiration, and tips en route to assist with carrying out new mediations for long haul achievement and way of life change. Discoveries from a pilot study directed at the Miriam Clinic's Weight Control and Diabetes Exploration Center show that fat people taking part in a get-healthy plan that was upheld by an expert Wellbeing Mentor or companion lost clinically huge measures of weight (i.e., no less than 5% of their underlying body weight)

Wellbeing Mentors offer an unexpected component in comparison to treatment or guiding in that training assists clients with shaping an objective situated point of view. Directing can assist people with zeroing in on critical thinking and helping a pessimistic inclination, circumstance, or damaging issue. Training is intended to work WITH the client in recognizing objectives and pursuing the objectives in a commonly upheld way. Mentors can offer everyday help and inspiration to assist people with remaining focused and gain ground toward their objectives. Instructing includes giving people an additional component and push to arrive at their objectives.

Looking for help from a certified psychological wellness expert may be the answer for some normal counting calories issues and weight the board battles. Goad Wellbeing endeavors to acquaint a far reaching approach with assisting clients with finding the genuine purposes for bombed endeavors at rolling out enduring improvements for health concerns. At Chafe Wellbeing, heftiness and different issues are seen as a clinical issue and hence, are treated with proof based, clinical intercessions. Infuriate Health offers both guiding mediations, as well as instructing bundles accessible for up close and personal meetings or online virtual meetings.

CHAPTER 12: OVERSEEING HESITANCE AND DISAPPOINTMENTS

Making Plans For Defeating Enticements And Wants

You would concur that surrendering to enticement when on a careful nutritional plan is a vibe that is undoubtedly intimately acquainted for the vast majority.

We go out to eat with companions, we go to a family birthday festivity, or our housemate forgot about a pizza on the counter with a sign on the crate that expresses "Free to a Decent Home".

Anything that the reason, we yield to these allurements and undermine our eating regimen. We indulge at eateries, or we conclude that yes we will have the enormous cut of cake at the birthday celebration.

That free pizza on the counter?

No one simply eats one cut of pizza. Isn't that so? Right.

Tragically, these snapshots of shortcoming dial us back on our excursion to our objective weight, and very much frequently one slip by turns into another, then another, until we are off our eating routine endlessly.

Indeed, even with the liberal and differed nature of a CSN diet program and enhancements, a large number of us actually find it undeniably challenging to settle on the best decisions with regards to adhering to our eating routine arrangement.

However, there is trust. Similarly as many individuals battle with defeating the compulsion to undermine their eating routine, so likewise many individuals have created different techniques for beating the allurement and remaining on their eating regimen. Here are a few fantastic focuses to contemplate whenever you are enticed to undermine your eating regimen.

1 Spotlight on Advantages

Beating enticement, similar to a significant part of the fat misfortune process, is about outlook. It is fundamental to modify how you see food, individual movement, and weight reduction overall.

As opposed to zeroing in on all the unfortunate however flavorful unhealthy food you are surrendering, you should modify your mentality to zero in on the solid decisions you are making all things being equal.

For instance, you can zero in on how the solid elective food sources you are eating are really great for you, how they are assisting you with assuming command over working on your general wellbeing, and that each quality food thing is assisting you with shedding abundance weight while cheering you look and into each day.

As a rule, that cut of cake looks significantly less mouth-watering in examination.

2 Add Scrumptious Fixings

Battling enticement frequently expects us to direct a little willful mental fighting.

One of the most outstanding ways of achieving this is to add better flavorings and garnishes to our quality food to assists us with hankering better dishes over unhealthy food. Different cooking styles, adding sauces we appreciate, or in any event, switching around the flavoring a little can take your protein and greens on a delightful excursion all over the planet.

Another strategy that functions admirably is utilizing a sluggish cooker to set up our food to stir things up a bit and add a few new flavors we probably won't have encountered previously.

Could do without broccoli? Quit steaming it and begin bubbling it with oil and garlic. Fed up with plain chicken or meat? Add some salsa, hot sauce, or fiery mustard. Cover your vegetables in herbed Greek yogurt sauce and Parmesan.

Search up certain recipes on the web, get new fixings, and get cooking. You will rapidly find that your allurements become less and farther between when you have better and more delectable options accessible.

3 Free Your Life of Triggers

What ignites your desires? What things in your day to day existence trigger those enticements? Everyone has triggers with regards to eating - individuals, spots, and sentiments that give us powerful urges to enjoy unfortunate low quality food gorging.

Time and again, we permit these triggers to bring us into gorging or eating in any event, when we aren't ravenous.

Assume command and free your life of these triggers where you work, live, and play. Any place you are encountering the most allurement, you really want to eliminate those triggers immediately.

On the off chance that specific companions or relatives who tend to urge you to indulge, don't eat feasts or go drinking with them.

You don't need to keep away from them inside and out, simply ensure that assuming they are a trigger impact for you that you pick non-food related exercises for your to share together.

As you kill triggers from your life, you will find that those allurements spring up definitely less every now and again than they used to.

4 Be Shrewd About Replacements in your eating regimen plan

One of the drawbacks to dispensing with triggers from your life is that it can prompt a general feeling of hardship.

As you attempt to kill those things from your eating routine that you know are triggers, you find it is increasingly hard to quit pondering them since you currently feel denied.

Accordingly, as you kill triggers from your life, begin tracking down better replacements for your number one tidbits and trigger food varieties. For instance, assuming that you are a pizza sweetheart, find a decent recipe that you appreciate for cauliflower-hull pizza.

This recipe cuts an enormous number of calories, carbs, and sugars from a dish you definitely realize that you will generally eat a greater amount of than you ought to. Assuming it's frozen yogurt you need, have a go at making frozen protein pops that are lower in sugar and carbs.

5 Increment Your Protein Admission

It is vital to consume lean protein with each dinner and bite, and you ought to never go longer than three hours during the day without eating something.

Lean protein contains less calories while encouraging your for longer timeframes than sugar rich snacks since protein takes more time to process.

Even better, protein really consumes more calories during processing, making it ideal for advancing that calorie shortfall you want to consume fat. As a matter of fact, for each 100 calories of protein you consume, 25 calories are consumed just to process and use the protein.

Get your protein at regular intervals, and you will find that your desires and enticements have started to evaporate increasingly more after some time.

6. Actually take a look at Yourself Prior to Eating

Most of health food nuts undermine their eating regimen when they aren't in the right outlook.

More often than not, individuals aren't even eager when they undermine their eating regimen, yet rather are adapting to feelings or stress. Solace food mitigates those sentiments, thus we frequently go to food to manage our sentiments.

Whenever you are feeling the requirement for some solace food, pause and do a fast self-assessment. Could it be said that you are really ravenous? Might you at any point hear or feel your stomach thundering?

No?

Then now is the ideal time to go accomplish something fun and useful that is non-food related until that desire to eat passes. Best calorie counters say it takes somewhere in the range of 2-10 minutes of positive interruption to conquer desires or allurement.

One more method that functions admirably is to hydrate to check whether your body is really ravenous or just enticed by solace food. Ordinarily individuals experience thirst like craving, and they find after a glass of cold water that they aren't exactly eager all things considered.

7 Hydrate

Each specialist you will at any point meet will suggest that you drink a lot of liquids, and in the event that you don't hydrate over the course of the day that you begin doing as such.

In addition to the fact that it is really great for your general wellbeing, yet it assists you with eating less, as well. Perhaps of the most ideal way you can battle the compulsion to undermine your eating regimen is to drink a tall virus glass of water. Water is non-fat, no-calorie, and important to support your life.

Individuals can go half a month without food, yet something like three days with no water. To sweeten the deal even further, drinking cold water consumes calories since your body needs to warm it up to utilize it. Standard hydration is most certainly key to conquering allurement when it strikes.

In conclusion, encountering enticement is a typical piece of changing your way of life to get thinner. Assuming that you never experienced allurement en route and everything easily fell into place for you, then, at that point, anybody would have the option to get more fit.

Commonly individuals set off on a weight reduction venture and don't understand the entirety of their terrible eating and way of life propensities until they begin to roll out an improvement.

Outfitting intellectually has an enormous effect in regards to long haul achievement or disappointment and figuring out how to conquer enticement as it very well may be a significant part of any drawn out health improvement plan.

With everything taken into account, you should choose to carry on with that better life and express no to your allurement. You should decide to eliminate those triggers from your life.

You should pursue those better decisions of what you eat and how you invest your energy.

Fat-misfortune won't occur without help from anyone else, and you can't arrive at your objective load without the important has a significant impact on in your mentality that will assist you with accomplishing what you have decided to do.

Make sure to zero in on the advantages of all that you are attempting to achieve with your better eating regimen and weight reduction. Your CSN diet plan goes quite far making your excursion more straightforward, yet that won't eliminate the day to day decision to adhere to your eating routine any less troublesome assuming you have an unfortunate attitude.

Change your reasoning, adjust your viewpoints about food and exercise, and remain focused on your CSN diet.

With time, persistence, and better decisions even the best of dietary enticements will ultimately fall away.

Recognizing Blunders And Using Them As Opportunities For Development.

We as a whole commit errors — it's simply aspect of being human. In any case, the main thing is the way we handle those missteps and how we gain and develop from them. This is the way you can move toward it in an engaging manner:

Own Ready: When you understand you've committed an error, the initial step is to recognize it. It's enticing to hide it away from view or shift the fault, yet assuming liability shows development and respectability. Along these lines, own ready, regardless of whether it's awkward.

Ponder What Turned out badly: Set aside some margin to contemplate what prompted the error. Was it a miscommunication, a mental blunder, or perhaps an absence of involvement? Understanding the main driver can assist you with trying not to misstep the same way later on.

Gain from It: Each slip-up is a chance to learn and develop. Thus, rather than harping on the negative, center around the examples you can detract from the experience. What might you at some point have done any other way? What will you do any other way sometime later? Embrace the opportunity to get to the next level.

Apologize if Important: Assuming that your misstep impacted others, make sure to. An earnest statement of regret can go quite far in fixing any put in a horrible mood or harmed connections. It shows that you're willing to get a sense of ownership with your activities and offer to set things straight.

Make Changes: Use what you've figured out how to roll out sure improvements in your methodology or cycles. Whether it's carrying out new methods, looking for extra preparation, or simply being more careful later on, find proactive ways to keep comparable mix-ups from reoccurring.

Look for Help: Make it a point to look for direction or backing from others, particularly in the event that you're feeling overpowered. At times, an external point of view can give significant bits of knowledge and assist you with exploring through testing circumstances all the more actually.

Pardon Yourself: At long last, make sure to be thoughtful to yourself. All of us are human, and we will undoubtedly commit errors occasionally. Thus, don't be too unforgiving with yourself. All things being equal, pardon yourself, gain from the experience, and push ahead with a reestablished feeling of assurance.

At last, it's not the slip-ups we make that characterize us — it's the means by which we decide to answer them. In this way, embrace your missteps as any open doors for development, and continue to endeavor to be simply the most ideal adaptation that you can be.

CHAPTER 13: RESPECTING YOUR PROSPERITY

Recognizing Your Achievements, Both On And Off The Scale

Pausing for a minute to perceive and praise your achievements, regardless of whether they're connected with your weight reduction venture, is so significant for remaining inspired and having a decent outlook on yourself. This is the way you can do it such that feels normal and human:

Recognize Your Advancement: It's not difficult to become involved with the numbers on the scale, yet make sure to likewise commend the more modest triumphs en route. Perhaps you've seen your garments fitting somewhat looser, or you have more energy to handle your day — that is progress worth celebrating!

Observe Non-Scale Wins: Progress isn't just about the numbers. Pause for a minute to recognize different accomplishments, such as going with better food decisions, hitting another individual best in your exercises, or essentially feeling more positive about your own skin.

Consider Your Excursion: Recall how far you've come since you began your excursion. Recollect the difficulties you've confronted and the obstructions you've survived. It's a demonstration of your solidarity and assurance, and you ought to be glad for yourself for the amount you've achieved.

Share Your Prosperity: Make sure to impart your victories to other people. Whether it's with companions, family, or your internet based local area, sharing your accomplishments can be engaging for both you and everyone around you. Besides, it's an incredible method for gathering together to celebrate and move others on their own excursions.

Indulge Yourself: You've really buckled down, so why not indulge yourself with something particularly amazing? Whether it's a spa day, another outfit, or a flavorful dinner at your #1 café, figure out how to remunerate yourself for your endeavors and commend your achievements such that feels significant to you.

Put forth New Objectives: Whenever you've praised your achievements, now is the right time to lay out new objectives to keep you propelled and centered. Contemplate what you need to accomplish straightaway and set reasonable, reachable focuses to pursue. Everything no doubt revolves around making a big difference for the energy and proceeding to challenge yourself.

Practice Appreciation: Pause for a minute to offer thanks for the headway you've made and the positive changes in your day to day existence. Being grateful for what you've achieved can assist you with remaining grounded and keen to your excursion, regardless of how far you actually need to go.

Keep in mind, your process is one of a kind to you, and each step in the right direction is something to be glad for. So find opportunity to praise your achievements, both of all shapes and sizes, and continue to push towards your objectives with certainty and assurance!

Sorting Out Some Way To Treat Yourself When You Achieve Objectives.

Treating yourself when you achieve objectives is a particularly incredible method for recognizing your diligent effort and praise your triumphs. Here are a sensible thoughts on how you can make it happen:

Enjoy Your #1 Feast: There's nothing very like partaking in a heavenly dinner to commend an unparalleled piece of handiwork. Whether it's indulging yourself with an extravagant supper at your number one eatery or preparing an extraordinary feast at home, get some margin to relish each chomp and partake in the occasion.

Plan a Loosening up Spa Day: Indulge yourself with a day of spoiling and unwinding at the spa. Book a back rub, a facial, or whatever other medicines that cause you to feel revived and invigorated. It's the ideal method for loosening up and re-energize after the entirety of your diligent effort.

Take a Smaller than usual Escape: Plan an end of the week escape to get away from the hurrying around of day to day existence. Whether it's a comfortable lodge in the mountains, a beachside retreat, or a pleasant city break, a difference in view can do ponders for your temperament and mentality.

Go a little overboard on Something You've Been Needing: Is there something you've been peering toward for some time however haven't gone a little overboard on yet? Whether it's another device, a piece of gems, or an extravagant thing for your house, this moment's the ideal opportunity to indulge yourself with something uniquely great as a prize for arriving at your objectives.

Have a Do-It-Yourself Spa Day at Home: In the event that you'd prefer stay in, why not make your own spa day at home? Run a loosening up bubble shower, light a few candles, and spoil yourself with your #1 skincare items. You might in fact toss on a comfortable robe and partake in a film long distance race subsequently for a definitive taking care of oneself day.

Put resources into Your Leisure activities: Indulge yourself with something that upholds your side interests or interests. Whether it's another book, workmanship supplies, or gear for your #1 game or movement, putting resources into things that give you pleasure can be a magnificent method for praising your accomplishments.

Plan a Great Action: Do something fun and energizing to commend your prosperity! Whether it's evaluating another experience like stone climbing or kayaking, taking a dance class, or basically going for a picturesque climb, pick a movement that causes you to feel invigorated and strengthened.

Have a Festival with Friends and family: Offer your accomplishments with loved ones by facilitating a festival or social event. Whether it's a little evening gathering, a patio grill, or an outing in the recreation area, encircling yourself with friends and family and offering your satisfaction to them can make the event much more exceptional.

Indulge Yourself with a Day of Unwinding: Go home for the day to just unwind and loosen up. Snooze, go through the day in your comfiest garments, and do anything causes you to feel cheerful and settled. Whether it's perusing a book, going for a comfortable stroll, or marathon watching your #1 Network program, allow yourself to partake in some merited rest and unwinding.

Just Partake in the Occasion: At times, the most effective way to treat yourself is to just partake in the sensation of achievement and relax at the time. Take a full breath, consider how far you've come, and permit yourself to feel pleased with all that you've accomplished. You've buckled down, and you have the right to commend your outcome in the manner feels generally significant to you!

Keep in mind, treating yourself is tied in with recognizing your accomplishments and carving out opportunity to see the value in all the difficult work you've placed in. So feel free to praise your outcome such that feels ideal for you — whether it's large or little, excessive or straightforward, mainly, it gives you pleasure and joy!

Committing To A Happier, Healthier Lifestyle Long-term

Committing to a happier, healthier lifestyle for the long term isn't just about making a temporary change—it's about embracing a mindset and habits that will benefit you for years to come. Here's how you can approach it in a relatable way:

Know Your Why: Start by understanding why you want to make these changes. Whether it's to feel more energetic, be there for your loved ones, or simply live a more fulfilling life, knowing your motivations can help keep you focused when things get tough.

Take Small Steps: Rome wasn't built in a day, and neither is a healthier lifestyle. Instead of trying to overhaul everything at once, focus on making small, sustainable changes that you can stick with over time. Maybe it's swapping out sugary drinks for water, or taking a short walk every day—whatever feels manageable for you.

Find What Works for You: There's no one-size-fits-all approach to health and happiness. Experiment with different strategies—whether it's yoga, running, meal prepping, or meditation—and see what resonates with you. The key is to find activities and habits that you enjoy and that fit into your lifestyle.

Be Kind to Yourself: Change is hard, and it's normal to have setbacks along the way. Instead of beating yourself up when things don't go as planned, practice self-compassion. Treat yourself with the same kindness and understanding that you would offer to a friend who's struggling.

Focus on Progress, Not Perfection: It's easy to get caught up in the idea of being perfect, but the truth is, nobody is. Instead of striving for perfection, focus on progress. Celebrate the small victories—the days when you choose a salad over a burger, or the mornings when you make it to the gym—even if they seem insignificant.

Build a Support System: Surround yourself with people who support your goals and cheer you on along the way. Whether it's friends, family, or online communities, having a support system can make all the difference when it comes to staying motivated and accountable.

Prioritize Balance: Remember that health isn't just about what you eat or how much you exercise—it's about finding balance in all areas of your life. Make time for hobbies, relationships, and relaxation, and don't forget to indulge in the occasional treat or indulgence.

Stay Flexible: Life is unpredictable, and it's important to be flexible in your approach to health and happiness. If something isn't working, don't be afraid to pivot and try something new. The key is to keep experimenting and learning what works best for you.

Celebrate Your Wins: Finally, don't forget to celebrate your successes along the way. Whether it's reaching a milestone on your fitness journey, hitting a new personal best, or simply feeling more energetic and alive, take a moment to pat yourself on the back and acknowledge how far you've come.

By approaching your journey to a happier, healthier lifestyle with patience, kindness, and flexibility, you can create lasting change that enriches your life in countless ways. Remember, it's not about perfection—it's about progress, and every step you take brings you closer to the life you want to live.

Chapter 14: Sustaining Your Advancement Over Time

Making The Shift From Weight Reduction To Maintenance

While losing weight is difficult for many people, it is even more challenging to keep the weight off. Most people who lose a large amount of weight have regained it 2 to 3 years later. One theory about regaining lost weight is that people who decrease the amount of calories they consume to lose weight experience a drop in the rate their bodies burn calories. This makes it increasingly difficult to lose weight over months. A lower rate of burning calories may also make it easier to regain weight after a more normal diet is resumed. For these reasons, extremely low-calorie diets and rapid weight loss are discouraged.

Losing no more than 1/2 to 2 pounds per week is recommended. Incorporating long-term lifestyle changes is needed to increase the chance of successful long-term weight loss.

Weight loss to a healthy weight for a person's height can promote health benefits. These include lower cholesterol and blood sugar levels, lower blood pressure, less stress on bones and joints, and less work for the heart. It is vital to maintain weight loss to obtain health benefits over a lifetime.

Keeping extra weight off takes effort and commitment, just as losing weight does. Weight loss goals are reached by a combination of changes in diet, eating habits, and exercise. In extreme circumstances, people turn to bariatric surgery.

Weight loss maintenance strategies

The strategies that encourage weight loss also play an important role in maintenance:

Support systems used effectively during weight loss can contribute to weight maintenance. According to the National Weight Control Registry, 55% of registry participants used some type of program to achieve their weight loss.

Physical activity plays a vital role in maintaining weight loss. Studies show that even exercise that is not rigorous, such as walking and using stairs, has a positive effect. Activity that uses 1,500 to 2,000 calories per week is recommended for maintaining weight loss. Adults should try to get at least 40 minutes of moderate to vigorous level physical activity at least 3 to 4 times per week.

Diet and exercise are vital strategies for losing and maintaining weight. Ninety-four percent of the registrants in the National Weight Control Registry increased their physical activity.

Once the desired weight has been reached, the gradual addition of about 200 calories of healthy, low-fat food to daily intake may be attempted for one week to see if weight loss continues. If weight loss does continue, additional calories of healthy foods may be added to the daily diet until the right balance of calories to maintain the desired weight has been determined. It may take some time and record keeping to determine how adjusting food intake and exercise levels affect weight. A nutritionist can help with this.

Continuing to use behavioral strategies is necessary for maintaining weight. Be aware of eating as a response to stress. Also, use exercise, activity, or meditation to cope instead of eating.

A temporary return to old habits does not mean failure. Paying attention to dietary choices and exercise can help maintain weight loss. Identifying situations, such as negative moods and interpersonal difficulties, and using alternative methods of coping with such situations rather than eating can prevent returning to old habits.

Weight cycling

Weight cycling is losing and regaining weight multiple times. Some studies suggest that weight cycling, also called "yo-yo dieting," may result in some health risks. These include high blood pressure, gallbladder disease, and high cholesterol. However, these studies are not true for everybody. The best strategy is to avoid weight cycling and maintain a healthy weight through a commitment to increased physical activity and healthy eating.

One myth about weight cycling is that a person who loses and regains weight will have more difficulty losing weight again and maintaining it compared to a person who has not gone through a weight-loss cycle. Most studies show that weight cycling does not affect the rate at which the body burns fuel. Also, a previous weight cycle does not influence the ability to lose weight again. In addition, weight cycling does not increase the amount of fat tissue or increase fat distribution around the stomach.

Techniques For Avoiding Relapse And Maintaining Focus

Avoiding setbacks and staying focused on your health goals is no easy feat, but here are some down-to-earth strategies that can help:

Know Your Triggers: Take some time to recognize what tends to throw you off track. Whether it's stress, boredom, or certain situations, identifying your triggers can help you anticipate challenges and develop effective coping strategies.

Find Healthy Coping Mechanisms: Instead of turning to unhealthy habits when you're stressed or upset, find healthier ways to cope. Whether it's going for a walk, talking to a friend, or practicing deep breathing exercises, having alternative coping mechanisms can help you stay on course.

Stay Present: Mindfulness can be a powerful tool for maintaining focus. Try to stay present in the moment, paying attention to your thoughts, feelings, and behaviors. This can help you recognize when you're veering off track and make conscious choices to stay aligned with your goals.

Set Clear Boundaries: Establish clear boundaries around your health goals. This might involve setting rules for yourself, such as limiting certain foods or activities that are triggers for unhealthy behaviors. Having clear boundaries can help you stay accountable and focused.

Build a Support Network: Surround yourself with people who support your health goals and encourage your progress. Whether it's friends, family, or online communities, having a support network can provide motivation, accountability, and encouragement when you need it most.

Celebrate Progress: Don't forget to celebrate your successes along the way, no matter how small. Recognize and acknowledge the progress you've made, and give yourself credit for your efforts. Celebrating your wins can help keep you motivated and focused on your goals.

Stay Flexible: Be willing to adapt your strategies as needed. Life is full of unexpected twists and turns, so it's important to be flexible and open-minded. If something isn't working, don't be afraid to try a different approach.

Practice Self-Compassion: Be kind to yourself, especially when things don't go as planned. Remember that setbacks are a natural part of any journey, and beating yourself up over them won't help. Treat yourself with the same compassion and understanding that you would offer to a friend.

Stay Consistent: Consistency is key when it comes to maintaining focus on your health goals. Commit yourself to prioritizing your well-being every day, even when life gets busy or challenging.

Stay Positive: Finally, maintain a positive outlook and mindset as you work towards your goals. Focus on what you can control, and approach challenges with optimism and resilience. Remember that setbacks are temporary, and every small step forward brings you closer to your ultimate goal.

By incorporating these strategies into your daily life, you can avoid relapse and stay focused on your health goals, even when faced with challenges or setbacks. Remember, progress takes time, so be patient with yourself and keep moving forward one step at a time.

CONCLUSION: YOUR PATH TO A HEALTHIER LIFESTYLE

Considering The Lessons You've Learned And The Adjustments You've Made.

Reflecting on the lessons learned and adjustments made throughout your health journey is key to staying on track and continuing to progress. Here's how you can approach this reflection in a relatable way:

Celebrate Your Progress: Take a moment to acknowledge how much you've grown and achieved since you began your health journey. Whether it's losing weight, improving your fitness, or adopting healthier habits, celebrate the milestones you've reached and the progress you've made.

Learn from Challenges: Reflect on the challenges you've faced along the way. Maybe you struggled with cravings, faced setbacks, or found it difficult to stay motivated at times. Take the opportunity to learn from these challenges and consider what you can do differently in the future.

Adjust Your Approach: Based on your reflections, think about how you can adjust your approach moving forward. Maybe you need to set more realistic goals, find new ways to cope with stress or seek support from others. Be open to making changes and trying new strategies to help you succeed.

Find What Works for You: Take note of the habits and strategies that have been most effective for you. Whether it's meal prepping, scheduling regular workouts, or practicing mindfulness, identify what works best for your lifestyle and personality.

Stay Positive: Focus on the positives of your journey, even when faced with challenges. Instead of dwelling on setbacks, remind yourself of how far you've come and the progress you've made. Stay positive and keep moving forward, one step at a time.

Celebrate Small Wins: Don't underestimate the power of small victories. Whether it's choosing a healthy snack over junk food or completing a challenging workout, celebrate every accomplishment along the way. These small wins add up and help keep you motivated.

Be Kind to Yourself: Remember to be kind to yourself throughout your journey. Nobody is perfect, and it's okay to have setbacks or bad days. Treat yourself with compassion and understanding, and don't be too hard on yourself when things don't go as planned.

By taking the time to reflect on your health journey, you can gain valuable insights that will help you stay focused and motivated as you continue to work towards your goals. Remember that progress takes time, and every step forward, no matter how small, is a step in the right direction. Keep believing in yourself and the progress you've made so far.

Resolving To Pursue Ongoing Development And Personal Advancement

Deciding to keep growing and advancing personally is a big step toward a more fulfilling life. Here's how you can express this idea in a relatable way:

Keep Learning: Life is full of opportunities to learn new things, whether it's picking up a new hobby, exploring different cultures, or diving into a subject you've always been curious about. Embrace these chances to expand your knowledge and understanding of the world around you.

Set Meaningful Goals: Take the time to think about what you want to achieve in different areas of your life—whether it's your career, relationships, health, or personal development. Set goals that resonate with you and align with your values, and then take consistent steps toward making them a reality.

Step Out of Your Comfort Zone: Growth often happens when we push ourselves beyond what feels safe and familiar. Don't be afraid to take risks and try new things, even if they feel intimidating at first. You might be surprised by what you're capable of accomplishing.

Reflect on Your Progress: Now and then, take a moment to look back on how far you've come. Celebrate your achievements and milestones, no matter how small, and acknowledge the obstacles you've overcome along the way. This can help you stay motivated and inspired to keep moving forward.

Stay Open-Minded: Keep an open mind to new ideas, perspectives, and experiences. Be willing to listen to others, even if their opinions differ from your own, and be curious about the world around you. You never know what you might discover or how it might change your life for the better.

Practice Self-Improvement: Invest in yourself by prioritizing activities and practices that promote your personal growth and well-being. Whether it's taking care of your physical health, nurturing your relationships, or cultivating a positive mindset, make self-improvement a priority in your life.

Surround Yourself with Support: Surround yourself with people who believe in you and support your goals. Whether it's friends, family, mentors, or colleagues, having a strong support system can provide encouragement, guidance, and accountability as you work toward your aspirations.

Be Patient with Yourself: Remember that personal growth is a journey, not a destination. It's okay to take things one step at a time and progress at your own pace. Be patient with yourself, and trust that with time and effort, you'll continue to evolve and flourish in meaningful ways.

By committing to ongoing personal development, you're investing in your happiness, fulfillment, and success. Embrace the journey ahead with enthusiasm and determination, and never stop striving to become the best version of yourself.

Motivating People To Set Out On Their Path To Improved Health

Motivating others to begin their journey towards improved health is all about connecting with them on a personal level and inspiring them to take that first step. Here's how you can do it:

Share Your Story: Start by sharing your own experiences with health and wellness. Whether you've struggled with weight, overcome health challenges, or simply made positive changes in your lifestyle, sharing your journey can inspire others to believe in their ability to change.

Focus on Progress, Not Perfection: Encourage people to focus on progress rather than perfection. Remind them that every small step they take towards better health is a step in the right direction and that setbacks are a natural part of the process.

Offer Support and Encouragement: Let people know that they're not alone on their journey to better health. Offer your support, encouragement, and guidance every step of the way, and remind them that you believe in their ability to succeed.

Provide Practical Tips: Offer practical tips and advice to help people get started on their journey. Whether it's meal prep ideas, workout suggestions, or stress management techniques, providing actionable advice can help people feel more confident about making positive changes.

Highlight the Benefits: Talk about the many benefits of living a healthy lifestyle, such as increased energy, improved mood, better sleep, and reduced risk of chronic disease. Help people understand how prioritizing their health can improve every aspect of their lives.

Lead by Example: Be a role model for healthy living by practicing what you preach. Show others that living a healthy lifestyle is not only possible but enjoyable and rewarding. Share your healthy habits and choices to inspire others to follow suit.

Create a Supportive Community: Foster a supportive community where people can connect with others who are on a similar journey. Whether it's through social media groups, fitness classes, or local meetups, creating a sense of community can provide invaluable support and motivation.

Celebrate Achievements: Celebrate the achievements and milestones of those who are working towards better health. Whether it's losing weight, hitting a fitness goal, or making positive changes to their diet, acknowledge their progress and celebrate their successes.

Encourage Persistence: Remind people that change takes time and that it's normal to face challenges along the way. Encourage them to stay persistent, stay positive, and keep moving forward, even when the going gets tough.

Emphasize Self-Care: Stress the importance of self-care as a fundamental part of a healthy lifestyle. Encourage people to prioritize activities that nourish their body, mind, and soul, such as getting enough sleep, practicing mindfulness, and spending time with loved ones.

By connecting with people on a personal level, offering practical advice, and providing ongoing support and encouragement, you can motivate them to take that first step towards improved health and wellness. Remember to lead by example, celebrate their achievements, and remind them that they have the power to transform their lives for the better.

Appendix: Sources of Ongoing Assistance

Tools For Monitoring Your Development And Creating New Objectives.

Here are some practical tools and strategies you can use to monitor your progress and set new objectives on your health journey:

Health and Fitness Apps: There are tons of great apps out there that can help you track various aspects of your health, like nutrition, exercise, sleep, and hydration. Apps like MyFitnessPal or Fitbit can be super helpful for keeping tabs on your daily habits and progress.

Journaling: Keeping a journal is a simple yet effective way to track your thoughts, feelings, and progress. You can jot down your achievements, setbacks, and any insights you gain along the way. Plus, it's a great way to reflect on your journey and set new goals.

SMART Goals: When setting new objectives, it's important to make them SMART: Specific, Measurable, Achievable, Relevant, and Time-bound. This helps you create clear, actionable goals that you can track and work towards.

Progress Photos: Taking progress photos is a fantastic way to visually track your physical transformation over time. It's incredibly motivating to see how your body changes as you make progress towards your goals.

Body Measurements: Keeping track of measurements like weight, waist circumference, body fat percentage, and muscle mass can give you a more comprehensive view of your progress. You can use these metrics to make adjustments to your plan and stay on track.

Fitness Assessments: Regularly assessing your fitness level is key to monitoring your progress and setting new goals. Simple tests like counting push-ups or measuring your mile time can give you concrete benchmarks to work towards.

Self-Assessment Tools: Tools like stress surveys, sleep trackers, and mood journals can help you evaluate various aspects of your health and well-being. This self-awareness can guide you in identifying areas for improvement and setting new objectives.

Feedback from Others: Don't be afraid to seek feedback from friends, family, or health professionals. Their insights can provide valuable perspectives and help you stay accountable to your goals.

Goal Tracking Apps: There are plenty of apps designed specifically for tracking goals and habits. These apps allow you to set goals, track your progress, and receive reminders to stay on track with your action plan.

Regular Reflection: Finally, make time for regular reflection on your progress and goals. Take a step back to consider what's working, what's not, and what you want to focus on next. This reflection is essential for staying motivated and continuing to move forward on your health journey.

By using these tools and strategies to monitor your development and set new objectives, you can stay focused, motivated, and accountable as you work towards your health goals. Remember to be patient with yourself, celebrate your progress, and keep pushing towards a healthier you

RECIPES AND MEAL IDEAS TO KEEP YOU INSPIRED IN THE KITCHEN

Breakfast Treats:

Serve fluffy scrambled eggs over whole-grain bread with sautéed spinach, mushrooms, and feta cheese.

Smooth avocado toast with cherry tomato slices, red pepper flakes, and a balsamic glaze drizzle.

Blended berries, banana, spinach, almond milk, chia seeds, and granola for crunch make up this energizing smoothie bowl.

A dollop of Greek yogurt and fresh berries accompany these banana-oat pancakes, which are made with mashed banana, oats, eggs, and a pinch of cinnamon.

A whole-grain tortilla encases a smoked salmon and avocado breakfast burrito topped with scrambled eggs, salsa, and spinach.

For a tropical twist, try a Greek yogurt parfait covered with honey, sliced almonds, and diced mango or pineapple.

Lunch Ideas:

A vibrant salad with a Mediterranean flair that includes cucumber, cherry tomatoes, feta cheese, Kalamata olives, mixed greens, and a vinaigrette made with herbs and lemon.

hummus, shredded carrots, cucumber, lettuce, and a splash of fresh lemon juice are all included in this veggie-packed wrap made of turkey or tofu.

A filling bowl of quinoa, black beans, avocado slices, roasted sweet potatoes, and a creamy tahini sauce is served in this Buddha bowl.

Accompanied by crisp whole-grain bread, a caprese salad features juicy tomatoes, fresh mozzarella, basil leaves, and a balsamic sauce.

Bell peppers filled with quinoa and black beans, garnished with fresh cilantro and melted cheese and accompanied by guacamole on the side.

Lettuce wraps with tuna or chickpea salad, chopped cucumber, shredded carrots, and a squeeze of lemon juice.

Ideas for Dinner:

Honey-balsamic glaze-drizzled sweet potatoes and roasted Brussels sprouts accompany the grilled lemon-herb chicken.

Serve spicy shrimp over brown rice or cauliflower rice, tossed with bell peppers, snap peas, broccoli, and a zesty ginger-garlic sauce.

Serve this tasty vegetarian curry over basmati rice or naan bread. It is made with tomatoes, spinach, and aromatic spices and cooked in coconut milk.

Wild rice pilaf and roasted Brussels sprouts are served over baked salmon glazed with a maple-mustard mixture.

A savory blend of quinoa, sautéed kale, cranberries, and pecans is stuffed into vegetarian acorn squash and drizzled with tahini dressing.

With aromatic spices and a creamy tomato-based sauce, basmati rice and naan bread are served alongside chicken or tofu tikka masala.

Filling Snacks:

Cinnamon-sprinkled whole-grain rice cakes with crunchy almond butter and banana slices.

A parfait of Greek yogurt topped with granola, honey, and fresh berries.

Crunchy vegetable sticks (carrots, celery, bell peppers) served with tzatziki dip or creamy hummus as a dip.

Dark chocolate chips, walnuts, almonds, and dried cranberries combine to create an energizing trail mix.
Snack: Ants on a log with celery sticks stuffed with cream cheese or nut butter and dusted with raisins or dried cherries.

Sea salt, garlic powder, and smoky paprika combine to create a flavorful and filling snack of crispy roasted chickpeas.

Nutritious Dessert Treats:

Warm-baked apples topped with a dollop of vanilla Greek yogurt and packed with walnuts, oats, and cinnamon.

For a gratifying sweet treat, try frozen banana slices or strawberries covered in dark chocolate.

A homemade version of chia seed pudding, flavored with vanilla essence and a hint of maple syrup, and served with coconut flakes or fresh fruit on top. Made using almond milk.

Blended frozen banana "nice cream" with cocoa powder and a small amount of almond milk, garnished with chopped almonds and shredded coconut.

Warm baked pear halves filled with oats, walnuts, honey, and cinnamon are served warm with a dollop of yogurt or vanilla ice cream.

Ripe avocados, cocoa powder, honey, and vanilla essence are mixed until smooth and creamy to make chocolate avocado mousse.

Winners of Meal Prep:

This vibrant, protein-rich quinoa salad is ideal for making in bulk and eating all week long. It includes roasted vegetables, chickpeas, and a zesty lemon-tahini vinaigrette.

Easy-to-assemble sheet pan fajitas including sliced chicken or tofu, onions, bell peppers, and Mexican seasonings, accompanied by whole-wheat tortillas and all the fixings.

For a convenient and wholesome lunch alternative, try mason jar salads stacked with roasted veggies, quinoa, grilled chicken or tofu, and a tangy vinaigrette.

Full of lean ground turkey, beans, tomatoes, and spices, slow cooker turkey chili is ideal for preparing in bulk and freezing for later use.

Made with eggs, sliced bell peppers, spinach, and feta cheese, these veggie-packed egg muffins bake up quickly for a quick breakfast or lunch.

GLOSSARY PAGE

Calories: This is a unit of measurement for the amount of energy in food and drink. Maintaining a record of your caloric consumption can aid in efficient weight management.

Macronutrients: Vital nutrients are required in high concentrations by the body for development and energy. Proteins, lipids, and carbs are the three primary macronutrients.

Carbohydrates: The nutrients that provide the body energy and are present in foods like bread, pasta, fruits, and vegetables. There are two types of carbs: complex carbohydrates (starches and fiber) and simple carbohydrates (sugars).

Proteins: Elements required for the synthesis of hormones and enzymes, as well as for the maintenance and repair of tissues. Meat, fish, poultry, eggs, dairy products, legumes, nuts, and seeds are all excellent sources of protein.

Fats: Highly concentrated energy sources that aid in the body's production of hormones and absorption of vitamins. Avocados, almonds, seeds, olive oil, fatty salmon, and coconut oil are good sources of fat.

Micronutrients: Vital nutrients, such as vitamins and minerals, that the body needs in smaller amounts.

Vitamins are organic substances with significant effects on immunity, metabolism, and general health. Many foods, including fruits, vegetables, whole grains, and lean meats, contain them.

Minerals are inorganic compounds that are necessary for several biological processes, such as neuron, fluid, and bone health. Foods high in minerals include dairy products, fortified cereals, nuts, and seeds, as well as leafy greens.

Fiber: A form of carbohydrate that the body is unable to digest, but which is crucial for maintaining blood sugar balance, gastrointestinal health, and weight control. Fruits, vegetables, whole grains, legumes, nuts, and seeds are good sources of fiber.

Antioxidants are substances that assist in shielding the body from harm brought on by dangerous chemicals known as free radicals. Dark chocolate, nuts, seeds, fruits, and vegetables are rich sources of antioxidants.

The process of keeping the body's fluid levels appropriate is known as hydration. Maintaining hydration is beneficial to general health and may aid in managing weight.

Whole foods are minimally processed foods that nonetheless have a high fiber and nutrient content. Fruits, vegetables, whole grains, lean meats, nuts, seeds, and legumes are a few examples.

Foods that have undergone cooking, refining, or ingredient addition that have changed from their natural condition are referred to as processed foods. Artificial chemicals, bad fats, and added sugars are common ingredients in processed foods.

Meal prep is the process of organizing and preparing meals ahead of time to reduce waiting times and encourage better eating practices. Preparing meals frequently entails preparing big quantities of food and dividing it into portions for later consumption.

Superfoods: Foods high in nutrients that are thought to be particularly advantageous for overall health and well-being. Berries, leafy greens, fatty fish, nuts, seeds, and entire grains are a few examples.

The process by which the body turns food and liquids into energy is called metabolism. Maintaining a healthy metabolism is crucial for both managing weight and general health.

Controlling portion sizes to avoid overindulging and preserve a healthy weight is known as portion control. Portion control is paying attention to serving sizes and cues from hunger and fullness.

Physical activity is any bodily movement that requires energy expenditure and advances fitness and health. Frequent exercise is essential for cardiovascular health, managing weight, and maintaining general well-being.